Praise for Pure Nurture: *A Holistic Guide to a Healthy Baby*

A wonderful and supportive guide for pregnancy. Pure Nurture: A Holistic Guide to a Healthy Baby is a fantastic resource with helpful exercises throughout the book and is sure to delight moms-to-be.

Margo Shapiro Bachman, MA, NAMA certified
Ayurvedic Practitioner and author of Yoga Mama Yoga Baby,
Ayurveda and Yoga for a Healthy Pregnancy and Birth

Pure Nurture is an invaluable resource for all mothers to be. Written from personal experience and with a gentle and selfless desire to demystify the full range of self-care options including: nutrition, mindfulness, yoga, movement, sleep, massage, and ways to optimize one's emotional safety net, Kristy Rodriguez's words provide a "GPS" – an easy to read map – for any woman considering pregnancy or doing her best to cherish and optimize the gift of pregnancy.

David Eisenberg, MD Adjust Associate Professor,
Harvard T.H. Chan School of Public Health Former
Founding Director of the Harvard Medical School
Division for Complimentary and Integrative Medicine

Brimming with valuable healthy tips, Pure Nurture: A Holistic Guide to a Healthy Baby is a clear, concise read that introduces concepts of Integrative Nutrition and applies them to the pregnancy journey, gently guiding mothers-to-be towards improved total wellness, including greater compassion for body, mind, and spirit.

Joshua Rosenthal, MScEd, Founder and
Director, Institute for Integrative Nutrition

Pure Nurture: A Holistic Approach to a Healthy Baby offers the tools all women need to cultivate a healthy baby and self - during pregnancy and beyond. A must read for all mothers-to-be!

Robynne Chutkan, MD, FASGE Integrative
gastroenterologist and author of Gutbliss, The
Microbiome Solution, and The Bloat Cure

Kristy Rodriguez is just the person to lead a mother-to-be through the transformative journey into parenthood. Including a special section on the practice of yoga and meditation during pregnancy, Pure Nurture: A Holistic Guide to a Healthy Baby is an empowering resource for the expectant mother. It will inspire her to choose a path of health and mindfulness, displaying the same kindness and nurturance toward herself as to her child and laying a strong foundation so that she may thrive in her new role as a parent.

Baron Baptiste, Author of New York
Times Bestseller; Perfectly Imperfect

Pure Nurture: A Holistic Guide to a Healthy Baby is an essential guide highlighting the benefits of yoga and mindfulness practices during pregnancy. Many find starting a personal practice intimidating, however, Kristy Rodriguez, an inspirational and compassionate guide, will help readers to create a personal practice using yoga and mindfulness during their pregnancy journey.

Rob Schware, Executive Director, The Give Back Yoga Foundation.

Kristy Rodriguez breaks the mold with this insightful, down-to-earth, and encouraging guide to maternal self care. If you're interested in learning how yoga, meditation, and other holistic practices can support your journey into motherhood, this book is for you. Filled with stories, practice guides, and poignant insights, this easy-to-read guide is a generous gift to parents everywhere.

Chelsea Roff, Founder and Director, Eat Breathe Thrive

Kristy is one of the most authentic and inspiring women I know. In her first book, Pure Nurture: A Holistic Approach to a Healthy Baby, she is deeply committed to helping pregnant women (or any woman!) understand and ultimately practice nourishment in all senses of the word. While it's so easy for a mother or mother-to-be to put her own needs on the back burner and get caught up in the daily demands of a growing family, Kristy inspires her reader to want to take care of herself first in order to be able to take care of others. Using her own real life experiences in an inviting way, Kristy shows us that self-care is not selfish but essential! From the advice on how to create a simple meditation practice amidst the chaos to how to carve out time to feed your body with nutrient-dense foods, it is evident that self-care is the road to health and happiness for a mama...and her entire family.

Elise Museles, Eating Psychology + Nutrition
Expert, Founder of Kale and Chocolate

This book is like a trusted advisor to consult with during one of the most transformative times in life. Kristy expertly yet practically guides you to find a successful path for a well-adjusted pregnancy journey. Highly recommended!

Mari Smith, Birth Doula and Founder of Celebrated Birth

Pure Nurture: A Holistic Guide to a Healthy Baby is a wonderful guide for women achieving their optimal pregnancy outcome by implementing important health and fitness resources and goals. Optimized health and physical activity improves your chances for the individual experience that you desire in pregnancy, labor and delivery. I have professionally known Kristy Rodriguez and feel most women would benefit from her own personal experiences in optimizing their health and overall-wellbeing.

Dr. Jack P. Ayoub, MD, FACOG, CEO and
President of Virginia Obstetrics & Gynecology.

"Kristy Rodriguez serves as a gentle, loving guide as she helps you achieve your healthiest pregnancy. Practical wisdom on every page makes this a must read for moms-to-be!"

Victoria Maizes, MD Executive Director, University of Arizona Center for Integrative Medicine. Author of Be Fruitful: The Essential Guide to Maximizing Fertility and Giving Birth to a Healthy Child.

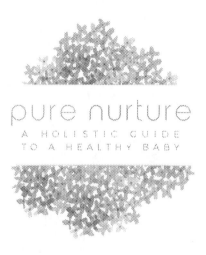

pure nurture

A HOLISTIC GUIDE
TO A HEALTHY BABY

By

Kristy S. Rodriguez

BALBOA.
PRESS

A DIVISION OF HAY HOUSE

Balboa Press books may be ordered through booksellers or by contacting:

Balboa Press
A Division of Hay House
1663 Liberty Drive
Bloomington, IN 47403
www.balboapress.com
1 (877) 407-4847

Print information available on the last page.

ISBN: 978-1-5043-6950-3 (sc)
ISBN: 978-1-5043-6951-0 (e)

Balboa Press rev. date: 02/07/2017

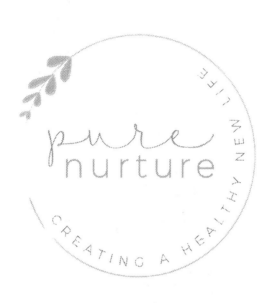

Dedication

To my husband, William, for his constant
encouragement and unconditional love.
To my two daughters, Eliana and Gabriela. You are
my inspiration and the reason this book exists.
&
To all mothers and mothers-to-be. May you radiate with the
love and care you have for yourself. May it flow over into the
lives of those around you, teaching the next generation to
be kind and compassionate to both themselves and others.

Self-care during pregnancy is the first gift
that the mother can give to her child.

—Mary Thompson,
"An Ayurvedic Approach to Prenatal Care"

Contents

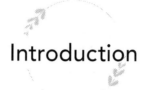

Introduction

Nourishing yourself in a way that helps you
blossom in the direction you want to go is
attainable, and you are worth the effort.

–Deborah Day

A miracle has occurred: you are creating a new life! Your body is now engaged in an incredible process during which, over the next forty or so weeks, you will experience new and different physical and emotional changes. If this is your first pregnancy, or even if it's your fourth, this one is unique to you. No two pregnancies are the same, no matter what people assume you'll feel because they felt it themselves. You can listen to the stories from your mom, sisters, and friends, but your story and your pregnancy are solely yours.

These next nine months are all about you and your growing baby. The fact that you have opened this book means that you are ready to take good (or even better) care of yourself and your baby. You know that your well-being has a direct effect on your developing baby, and you are willing to take time out of your busy life to focus on the larger picture of your pregnancy.

My goal for you as you read this book is that you learn new ways to feel your best, find more balance amidst all of the changes that are happening, and create a healthy foundation for your little one.

In his book *Magical Beginnings,* Deepak Chopra states, "From the moment of conception, the preborn baby experiences the thoughts and actions of her mother."[1] It's well-established by now that the mind and body are connected. When you are pregnant, your body and mind are also directly linked to the body and mind of your growing baby.

Caring for your baby includes caring for you. That's what this book is all about. Self-care is not a luxury, and it is not selfish. It is, in fact, vital to raising a child, who after all, will be completely dependent upon you for everything for years to come. So, as you read this, remember that these suggestions are meant to be helpful, not strident or judgmental. Do what you can, try what sounds interesting, and if you find something that works, then keep on doing it.

How to Use This Book

This book is a short and inspirational guide to support you through your pregnancy. It is dedicated to you. By providing you the tools needed to feel great, as well as tips on how to treat yourself and your baby with the love and respect you both deserve, this book can help you both be healthier throughout your journey together.

Whether you are trying to conceive, are already pregnant, or are now a mother to a brand new baby, this book will support you in learning new ways to practice essential self-care, habits that, once started, don't ever have to stop.

This book is <u>not</u> a medical guide. It is not meant to replace any medical advice from your doctor or midwife, nor is it a "things-I-must-do-in-order-to-be-a-good-person" guide. My intention is to provide you with support and share what inspired me during my own pregnancies to feel more comfortable in my own skin, in the hopes that you will feel encouraged to do more of what brings you joy and good health.

You can read this book from cover to cover or skip around. Take it with you wherever you go, or leave it on your nightstand for positive inspiration first thing in the morning or before you go to bed at night. When someone or something has put you through the wringer, or when you're craving that fifth doughnut of the day, grab this book and practice one of the tips that resonates with you the most.

Don't be afraid to write in this book—it is made especially for you. Highlight, underline, or make notes and doodles in the margins. At the end of each chapter, you will find space for journaling. Use this space to vent or to write a burst of inspiration or a short list of things you are grateful for that day. Some parts of this book will interest you more than others, so make a note of what you really like in order to quickly and easily find it again.

At the end of the book, you will find a link to a Self-Care Support Sheet. This is a summary sheet where you can write down the tools and tips that inspire you the most. A downloadable copy is also available on my website: purenurture.com/free-gifts. Print it out, fill it in, and hang it where you will see it often.

Send your friends to the website to get this tool too, because anyone (pregnant or not) can always benefit from a little self-care inspiration.

We all will sometimes get caught in a cycle of negative thoughts, and that's when practicing self-care is really important. You may still be thinking about all the things you have not done yet or all the things you have done "wrong" so far, like *gasp* that soft-serve ice cream cone you had last week or the latte from your favorite coffee shop. It's okay! You are okay and your baby is okay. So starting here and now, treat yourself with more love and respect. Let the past be in the past, because this is all about the right now. One of my favorite authors, Eckhart Tolle, sums it up beautifully: "Realize deeply that the present moment is all you ever have. Make the Now the primary focus of your life."[2]

Making time for self-care and creating the healthiest foundation possible for your growing little one is what makes a great mama. Together we will discover new ways you can have a happy, healthy, and more relaxed journey toward the birth of your baby.

Let us begin.

Journal Page

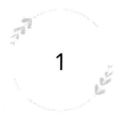

1

why self-care is important

The more successful you are in meeting your needs, the more likely you are to spend time in states of emotional comfort.
—Deepak Chopra, Magical Beginnings, Enchanted Lives

Self-care is the practice of actively ensuring your needs are met. The need for self-care is more important now than ever before, yet many of us have no idea of how to go about doing it. Our Western society, it seems, refuses to let us get off the hamster wheel. The rates of insomnia, depression, and anxiety in the US are off the charts. Self-care practices are not built into our society like they are into others, especially for prenatal and maternity care, and our habits are taking their toll on us.

David Ji, author and stress management expert, maintains that stress is how we respond when our basic human needs are not met.[3] He is not referring to trips to the spa or weekends away from it all; rather, he means the things we require every day, such as sleep and food. The best place to start taking care of yourself, then, is to ensure you are getting adequate rest and nourishment. By doing so, you can reduce the amount of stress hormones in your body, like cortisol, which have a direct effect on your growing baby. To put it plainly: the better you feel, the better your baby will feel.

Taking care of you means paying attention to YOUR needs before those of everyone around you. It requires a conscious decision to do so, which is why, in general, women will often do things for others at the expense of their own desires before they even think to question it. In reality, though, if you are mentally and physically depleted, it does not matter how much you want to do for others—you cannot do anything if you have nothing left to give. Your cup, so to speak, must be full before you can be the best version of yourself. Honor your needs first, and then, with a full cup, you will better support those around you. So, from now on, NEVER apologize for taking care of you.

This advice applies to everyone, but it is especially relevant during pregnancy, because your state of being will affect your baby. Stressors, as well as emotions like happiness and sadness, cause surges in various hormones. Having just determined that your baby experiences everything that you do, we can safely say that all of this has an effect on you both. "Science has demonstrated," states Deepak Chopra, "that every wisp of experience is metabolized into the substance of our minds and bodies, both before and after we are born into this world."[4] It is safe to conclude, then, that self-care is not only good for you, it is also good for your baby.

Addressing your needs before those of others is about more than just taking care of your physical self. Your spiritual and emotional self often goes untended to and is, therefore, in need of even more nourishment and respect. To address this imbalance, some people meditate, some make time to read a book, and others workout. There is no one way to feed your spirit; sometimes, as it happens, the simplest actions are often the ones that have the greatest effects.

For example, on a visit to my hometown, I called my friend, Maggie (not her real name), to see if she would like to grab a late dinner. It was already late, so I wasn't sure if she would be available, but I called anyway because getting food with a good friend that night was my attempt at self-care.

Maggie's response to my invitation was, "Ah, um, well, normally I don't say this, and I hate to say it, but um, no, I can't. I'm going to hang with my hubby tonight. I've been away for three nights and…" She continued on, explaining herself and apologizing. I could feel her distress and guilt over saying no.

My response to her was, "It's absolutely okay! Please don't feel bad. It was a last-minute call. Have a great time with your husband!" As bummed as I was not to see her, I was glad that Maggie was practicing her own self-care by honoring her needs in that moment.

After we got off the phone, I thought of all the times I have done exactly what she did: hemming and hawing and apologizing, unable to give a definitive "no" in a gentle and respectful way. The truth is, though, that it is absolutely okay to say no, and you do not have to apologize. Give your time and your energy the respect they deserve. Simply say: "No, I'm sorry, I can't. I would love to spend time with you, but I have _____ to do. Let's definitely make plans for another time!" And you could add, "Thanks for thinking of me! It means a lot that you want to spend time with me." Most people will understand; as for the ones who may have a problem with it... well, that is their issue, and it has nothing to do with you.

Sometimes you might feel like you do not have a legitimate reason for saying no, because the only one you have is that you are just too tired. But, guess what? That IS a legitimate reason! Even more so when you're pregnant. "Sorry, I can't go out tonight. This bun in the oven makes me sleepy, and I am going to bed early. You have fun, though, and thanks for the invite!"

When you approach decisions from this perspective, from a place where you are making them out of love for yourself and your happiness rather than out of guilt, you are practicing the best kind of self-care. You will feel confident and content with your decision to make yourself your priority. On the other hand, when you say yes out of guilt or a feeling of obligation to someone, that is when resentment (both toward yourself and others) builds. Release the grip of guilt and doing things out of obligation, and your life will change for the better.

Having a self-care practice for your entire life will help you maintain a state of ease. You will more quickly and easily let go of tension and constriction in your body. Knowing that life is an ever-changing plain (especially when you become a parent), having a cache of self-care habits will help you ride the waves of life more confidently, allowing you to quickly find a state of balance when the ups and downs occur.

We cannot protect our babies or ourselves from every upsetting thing in life. You feeling your best ultimately creates the best possible environment within which your baby can grow. Treat yourself (body and mind) and your baby with kind-heartedness, compassion, and unconditional love. You both deserve it.

Journal Page

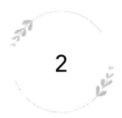

2

nutrition and nourishment

Honor the physical temple that houses you by
eating healthfully, exercising, listening to your body's
needs, and treating it with dignity and love.
—Wayne Dyer, The Invisible Force

Nutrition and nourishment are not just about what you eat, but also how you eat, no matter where you are in life. This topic is near and dear to me, and I believe that it is incredibly important, so within these pages we will dive deeply into this subject matter.

As a graduate of the Institute for Integrative Nutrition, I learned from Joshua Rosenthal, its founder, about what he calls "Primary Food" and "Secondary Food." Primary Food is more than what is on your plate; it is the "life food," the things that feed us on both the emotional and spiritual levels. Secondary Food is the actual food that we chew and swallow, nourishing us on a physiological level.[5] Both types of nourishment are essential for a balanced and healthy life.

Most pregnant women worry more about the actual food they are or are not eating, so let us put the primary food aside for the moment and, first, talk nutrition.

It is indisputable that pregnancy is one of the most important times in your life, and that incorporating healthy eating into your diet is essential. Nutrition matters not only for yourself but for your growing baby as well. The vast amounts of information about what you should and should not eat can make the discussion of nutrition feel overwhelming. Rather than pile on with statistics, facts, and fear-based information, we are going to take a look at this topic from a different angle: Nutrient Density.

Nutrient-Density is a food's measurement of nutrients (vitamins, minerals, etc.) in relation to its number of calories. The more nutrient-dense a food is, the more bang for your buck it provides, so to speak. Given that we are inundated every day with differing opinions on which foods are "best" for you, your body type, and your lifestyle, I believe that focusing on nutrient density is the most straightforward path toward healthy eating.

There are few other times in life when the quality of your food is more important than it is during pregnancy. In 2014 researchers from the Center for Chemical Regulation and Food Safety analyzed eleven studies and found that higher birth weights, which are associated with better brain development during later years, are linked to the amount of fruits and vegetables a mother eats during pregnancy. It also showed that improving the quality of food a woman eats is more effective than just increasing the quantity.[6]

How nutritious/nutrient dense is your food? Here are some quick and easy questions to help you decide: How close is your food to the source it was taken from— ground, garden, or farm? How much packaging was used before it got to you? How closely does it resemble its most natural form? The health value of your food is closely related to how close it is from its origins. Fresh fruits and veggies from the local farmer's market are great; potato chips and fruit cakes are not as good. As Michael Pollan, author of *Food Rules*, wrote, "If it came from a plant, eat it; if it was made in a plant, don't."[7]

I realize that not everyone around the country has access to the same resources, but if you are able to buy organic, do. Most grocery stores now carry good selections of organic and fresh(er) foods. Take a moment to also read the Environmental Working Group's Dirty Dozen, a list of the twelve fruits and vegetables containing the most pesticides and harmful chemicals. If you can only get a few organic items, the ones on this list would be the best place to start.[8]

Being selective about certain foods is worthwhile in order to avoid the chemicals commonly used on their nonorganic counterparts. For example, due to their fragile skin and delicate growing conditions, conventional strawberries may contain large amounts of pesticides and chemicals to help them grow. So, if you were to choose one organic item to buy, this should be a prime contender. On the other hand, buying organic is not terribly important for certain foods, like avocados or pineapples, because they have thick skins that you cut off and discard (the skins of fruits and vegetables are where most pesticides and residues are found). Avocados are on the Environmental Working Group's Clean Fifteen list because only 1% of all avocado samples showed any detectable pesticides. To read the full list of "clean" and "dirty" foods, visit their website: ewg.org.[9]

Your Relationship with Food

Before I delve deeper into healthy food choices, I first want to share a story of my relationship with food. In my first year of college, I felt out of control of, and insecure about, myself. Food became my crutch—it was the one thing I could easily control. My focus at that time was on how many grams of fat and the number of calories I was consuming. To stay on track, I ate mostly processed foods so that I could easily read the labels on the packages and keep a detailed record of the limited fat grams and calories I was allowing myself to eat. My self-imposed limit was no more than five grams of fat a day. This was also the time in the 1990s when low-fat and non-fat foods were the latest focal points of the diet craze.

After a few years of this controlled and limited diet, my body could no longer maintain its restrictive ways, and the pendulum swung in the opposite direction. I began binge eating. I would buy a large package of candy or a pint of Ben and Jerry's ice cream and finish it off in one sitting. After several years of this compulsive eating, I gained about thirty pounds. As I noticed my weight gain, I tried to restrict my fat and calorie intake, just like I had done in college, but instead of finding success, I found that I could no longer maintain such a strict and limited diet. I would binge the day after restricting, and thus the compulsive eating would continue.

Then, in my early twenties, I found myself in a position I never thought I would get into: with my head hung over the toilet, purging all the food I had just engulfed. I knew that I needed help, and in that moment I knew that I was completely ready to accept it.

I spent a few years with a dietician who specialized in eating disorders and many subsequent years with a therapist. I learned from them that my eating disorder wasn't really about the food but about issues of control and how that defined my sense of self-worth and feelings of success. I would progress, take steps back (relapse), make more progress, and eventually I took fewer steps back. This process lasted a few years, until one day when I realized that I was no longer obsessed with what, when, and how much I was eating. It had been over six months since I had binged or purged; then six months turned into a year, and so on and so forth. It has now been over twelve years since I recovered from my eating disorder.

I share this story with you because I want you to know that if you are dealing with, or have dealt with, food or body image issues, you are not alone. Even if you have never had a fully developed eating disorder, you or someone you know may have experimented with dieting or felt concerned about weight or body shape. I also use this story as a precaution, because pregnancy can reactivate negative thoughts about food and body weight, and it may feel scary to realize that your body is going to change in ways it never has before. I am here to tell you that those changes are natural, and that by eating nurturing and nutritious foods, you may more easily accept that those changes are normal in the course of creating a new life. Instead of unhealthily obsessing over calories, you are now paying attention to what you eat for the right reason: your baby's health.

Making changes to your diet is a simple strategy if you think about it in this way: Seek out the colors of the rainbow in your fruits and veggies. Eat pure foods full of life-force energy, like fruits, veggies, organic dairy (I don't normally consume a lot of dairy products, however, I was obsessed with milk when pregnant), nuts, seeds, legumes, and whole grains. Limit your intake of foods that are devoid of this life-force energy, such as sugar, caffeine, highly spiced dishes, and food that has been fried, canned, or fermented. (It should be noted that leftovers, sadly, also fall into this latter category.)

Cravings and Aversions

What to do if you are totally on board with nutrient-dense eating, but you feel sick and do not want to eat at all? Every pregnancy is unique; however, it is normal that during the first three or four months (or more) you might find it especially hard to eat foods you like, let alone some you haven't always loved.

I know what that is like. During the seven months I spent trying to get pregnant, I imagined how healthily I would eat while pregnant. I thought about the foods I would enjoy and the ones I would cut out or avoid. I read books and researched about healthy eating during pregnancy. However, a few weeks after I saw those two pink lines on that little white stick, my fantasies of perfect eating flew right out the window.

I was nauseated almost every day during the first four months of both of my pregnancies. I felt an intense aversion to almost all foods, but especially toward vegetables and fruits. So much for my healthy eating plans. I found that between the nausea, exhaustion, and intolerance of certain smells, it was next to impossible to find something to eat. If the sight of a vegetable makes you want to vomit, I understand how you are feeling. I was once so focused on trying to eat healthily that I forced a steamed broccoli floret into my mouth and almost threw up on my plate right there in the middle of the restaurant. I could not even chew it.

The lesson I eventually learned was to be flexible and gentle with myself, especially during the first trimester. If you feel sick, do not force yourself to eat healthier just because it is what you think you should be doing. Being kind to yourself is equally as important to your developing baby as the food you are eating. And do not worry—your desire for food will eventually return… with a vengeance.

Feeling nauseated right now? This chart lists some go-to foods that are easy to eat and keep down. I have made some changes to the typical recommendations, providing you with the nutrient-dense versions that are also free of additives and artificial (and less-than-optimal) ingredients:

<u>Foods for Nauseated Moms-to-be</u>

Common Recommendations:	Nutrient-Dense Alternatives:
Saltine crackers	Whole wheat crackers (organic & non-GMO)
Ginger ale	Ginger tea (bag or fresh grated & strained ginger)

Popsicles (store bought with High Fructose Corn Syrup)	Homemade popsicles or store bought popsicles without added sugar, HFCS, or ingredients you cannot pronounce.
Peppermint star candies	Peppermint tea, peppermint leaves, peppermint essential oils (food-grade)
Yogurt with aspartame, food dyes or ingredients that you cannot pronounce.	Plain Greek yogurt (organic is best). Add honey or your own natural sweetener to taste.
White toast	Whole grain toast (check ingredient list, fewer is better)
Peanut butter	Any nut and seed butters (almond, peanut, cashew, etc.) Aim for fewer than 3 ingredients.

Other nutrient-dense foods known for their ability to ease nausea include: bananas, apples, lemon, nuts, and chicken broth.

A note on ingredients: When purchasing food in a package, the most important place to look in order to determine its quality is the ingredients list. Dr. Sears, a respected pediatrician and author of over forty books, recommends avoiding three ingredients: High Fructose Corn Syrup (HFCS or HFCS-90); hydrogenated oils; and anything with a number (such as food dyes, like Red Dye #40). By avoiding these three ingredients, you can eliminate over 90% of the junk food in your diet. If you would like to learn more, please visit: AskDrSears.com.[10]

As an added bonus, I have included a special chapter full of delicious, nutrient-dense snack ideas and recipes created by my good friend, eating psychology and health coach, Elise Museles, who is also the founder of Kale & Chocolate.

I find that discussions about food are immensely easier when it comes to sharing what we crave during pregnancy; it could, in fact, be an entire chapter unto itself. Cravings (and, conversely, aversions) may be the one topic where people feel free to express their true thoughts about eating without fear of judgment. It is important to explore the deeper meaning of cravings, because they can often mean much more than just "I want all the chocolate and fast food and candy I can get my hands on now that I have society's permission to eat all the time!"

Prior to my first pregnancy, I was a vegetarian for many reasons (ethical, dietary, etc.). Once I got pregnant, however, I had dreams about eating hamburgers. When I could stand it no longer, I gave in to the cravings and ate a hamburger for the first time in almost twenty years (twenty years!). Once I did, I soon experienced less fatigue and fewer sugar cravings. The results from a blood test later showed that I was anemic (low on iron). No wonder I was craving red meat! It was a good reminder to me to listen more to what my body is telling me, because it really does know best.

(One note about eating meat, especially during pregnancy: Aim for purchasing and consuming meat from trusted sources.

Look for local markets selling meat that has "Grass-Fed", "Green Fed" or "Pasture Raised" on the label.)

Dealing with cravings is not simply a matter of "yes" or "no" for everyone. If you struggle with whether or not to give into a craving, recognize that pregnancy is a completely different circumstance, and then ask yourself these two questions:

1. Am I thirsty? A common cause of cravings is simply a need for hydration. Drink a glass of filtered water and then check in with your craving or hunger level.

2. Is this craving due to a physical or emotional need? My need for iron-rich foods was due to my anemia, but sometimes we eat to suppress thoughts or feelings. An easy way to determine where the craving is coming from is to place one hand over your heart and one hand over your stomach. Close your eyes and ask yourself, "Am I actually hungry, or do I need something more than food?" If you sense that your craving is coming from an emotional need (your heart), try taking a warm bath, going for a walk or getting a hug from a loved one. This may satisfy what your body is craving. And at the end of the day, if you just really want something to snack on, go for it! Enjoy it thoroughly and completely. After all, everything in moderation leads to balance in, and enjoyment of, life.

One day I was watching a movie, and a woman in the film was eating a BLT (bacon, lettuce, and tomato sandwich). I do not eat bacon; in fact, I have not eaten it since I was a little girl, because I just do not like it. (For all you bacon lovers out there, I know, it is unfathomable.) Nor was I using mayonnaise on anything at that time. However, after weeks of nausea and food avoidance and aversion, that BLT looked delicious. I called my husband and asked him to pick up one for me on his way home.

"Are you sure?" he asked, knowing that he had never seen me eat a BLT before. After I assured him I was completely serious, he lovingly brought home the sandwich. As I took my first bite, I felt immense disappointment and irritation. "Honey... where is the mayo? There isn't any mayo on my BLT!"

Poor, sweet hubby... "But, mi amor, you don't eat mayo. I asked them to hold the mayo." With a sharp and agitated tone, I replied, "AND I DON'T EAT BACON! You can't have a BLT without mayo!"

My husband gave me one of those "are you kidding me?" looks, and I promptly ran upstairs to our bedroom and started sobbing. Raging pregnancy hormones that lead to embarrassing behavior aside, the moral of this story is to be explicit with your requests, and even text or write them out so that there is very little room for error. A pregnant woman's menu requests are nothing to mess with. Also, be as gentle as you can with your significant other, or any supportive friend or family member who is only trying to help you out, and you will be more likely to get what you ask for in the future.

Something I learned while studying to become a health coach that I have found exceedingly useful is the idea of "crowding out." It means you fill up on healthy things to, essentially, crowd out the foods that are not serving you. You focus on what you want to add in, thereby leaving less room for any food you are trying to avoid.

One of the best ways to crowd out is by drinking more water. Your blood volume will increase by 40% during pregnancy. Consuming enough water for your body is essential, especially since it aids in bolstering the amount of amniotic fluid surrounding your baby. By staying hydrated you will avoid common pregnancy ailments like constipation, urinary tract infections, and dry, itchy skin. Drinking water may even help prevent stretch marks (along with sesame seed or coconut oil belly rubs). Aim for eight 8-ounce glasses of water throughout the day. Drinking enough water can seem daunting and a little boring, not to mention the endless trips to the bathroom, but it really is worth it.

Most of us will find crowding out to be a challenge, because humans, in general, have a tendency to fixate on what we are trying to avoid. For example, if we are focusing on "not eating cookies," our brains ignore the word "not" and are left with "eating cookies." Think about how children behave when given directions—tell them not to do something and then they seem to do more of whatever it is. For example, "Don't run!" translates into "Run!" for some reason. Instead, you would say to a child, "Walk!" in order to get him or her to do what you want.

This insight into human nature was a light bulb for me, especially with my history of disordered eating. When I tell myself "you can't have this or that," or "from now on, no more chocolate," my brain goes into Ms. Rebellious mode, and suddenly all I can think about is what I have forbidden myself from consuming. Eventually my ability to resist fails, and I end up eating a large quantity of the forbidden food. If, however, I give myself permission to eat anything at any time, I know whatever it is I have obsessed over will always be there, that I can have some whenever I want, and then the desperation lessens.

Some tips to make it more interesting and enjoyable:

1. Keep a bottle with you at all times. Glass bottles are best (you avoid compounds that can leach from plastic water bottles). My favorite one is the Lifefactory bottle with a flip lid. (They offer a straw lid too, but this can cause you to swallow excess air, leading to excess gas and bloating.)

2. If you work at a desk during the day, keep a water pitcher and a glass on the desk next to you. You will end up sipping away during the day without even realizing it.

3. For a little treat, add a few tablespoons to a half cup fresh fruit juice to your water. It is a healthy alternative to soda.

4. Add fruit or veggie slices for a fun H_2O infusion. Some tasty options to consider are: orange, lemon, mint, cucumber, lime, and strawberry. Mix and match for fun flavors. It makes drinking water more enjoyable and adds a splash of nutrients, like vitamin C.

5. Try mineral water. When I was pregnant and feeling nauseated, cold mineral water was my go-to drink. I would mix it with my favorite fresh fruit juice (three parts water, one part juice).

Good nutrition does not have to be overwhelming. Just keep it simple, focus on nutrient-dense foods, and drink lots of water.

Journal Page

3

mindfulness and meditation

When a mother takes the time to quiet her mind and center herself, the calming physiological changes that are invoked through meditation are also communicated to the baby.
–Deepak Chopra, Magical Beginnings, Enchanted Lives

Mindfulness is usually referenced when discussing awareness of ourselves and our actions. It can also be used to discuss our eating behaviors and relationships with food. When you stop to consider what you are eating, you must also ask how, where, when, and why you are eating. In this section we will explore how eating in a relaxed state allows our bodies to absorb more of the nutrients from the food and leaves us feeling more satisfied in the end.

Think about a typical meal for you. Do you eat at your desk? While driving? While watching TV? If so, do you ever feel like your food is gone before you realized what and how much you were eating? These are factors that play a role in how your body accepts, assimilates, and digests food. Eating in front of the television is an especially dangerous behavior that essentially diverts our attention and prevents us from seeing our food. It can also easily lead to overeating, because we are not tuned in to the moment when our bodies signal they are full and satisfied.

To be more mindful of your mealtime behaviors, the first step is to sit down rather than standing at the counter or over the stove or at the refrigerator. (If you struggle with emotional eating of any kind, I recommend checking out one of my favorite books by Geneen Roth, *When You Eat at the Refrigerator, Pull Up a Chair.*)[11] Make mealtime an event by lighting a candle and turning on some soft music to create ambiance. Take three slow conscious breaths before eating, and then say a prayer, a blessing, or a thought of gratitude before you begin a meal. Eat slowly, savor the flavor, and chew thoroughly before swallowing.

A tasty way to practice mindful eating is the "chocolate meditation." If you do not want to use chocolate, you could practice with a small bite of any food. This specific meditation was adapted from the chocolate meditation originally posted on psychologytoday.com.[12]

Let's give it a try!

Choose some chocolate—either a type that you've never tried before or one that you have not eaten recently. Any kind will do, but the important thing is that it is a type you would not normally eat or that you do not often consume.

• Open the wrapper and inhale the aroma.

- Break off a piece and look at it. Really let your eyes drink in what it looks like, examining every nook and cranny.
- Set it on your tongue and close your mouth. Try to hold it on your tongue and let it melt, noticing any tendency to suck at it. Chocolate has over 300 different flavors. See if you can identify some of them.
- If you notice your mind wandering while you do this, simply notice where it went off to, and then gently bring it back to the present moment.
- After the chocolate has completely melted, swallow it very slowly and deliberately. Let it trickle down your throat.
- Repeat this with one other piece.

How was this different from the way you normally eat a piece of chocolate? Did the chocolate taste better than if you had simply eaten it at a breakneck pace? Do you feel more satisfied or satiated?

Aside from being an excellent excuse to consume chocolate, the purpose of this exercise is to demonstrate how eating slowly, methodically, and purposefully can be immensely satisfying.

Now, let us go beyond food and dive deeper into mindfulness and meditation. This is an example of primary food I mentioned, the food of life that nourishes heart and soul, the sustenance that is just as important as the actual food on your plate. Many people can easily identify what food is healthy, but they do not pay attention to what else they "feed" (or do not feed) themselves. Take a minute to contemplate the following: What fulfills you? What lifts your spirit? What energizes you? Calms you? Inspires you?

Next, think about the areas in your life where you might need extra nourishment. Perhaps it is time with friends and loved ones or time out in nature? Maybe it is making time for exercise, or fulfilling a professional or creative outlet? A creative way to determine the area(s) of your life that may need some extra attention is by doing a "Wheel of Life" activity.[13] Many life coaches implement this type of tool in their practices, and you can find a free downloadable version on my website: purenurture. com/free-gifts.

One of the simplest and most profound mindfulness practices is that of gratitude. Every day, think of one thing you are grateful for. It does not have to be something grandiose or complex. It can be as simple as, "I am grateful for this glass of clean water." There is research and science supporting the tangible benefits of having an attitude of gratitude. Research by UC Davis psychologist Robert Emmons, author of *Thanks! How the New Science of Gratitude Can Make You Happier*, shows that simply keeping a gratitude journal—regularly writing brief reflections on moments for which we are thankful—can significantly increase our well-being and overall satisfaction with life.[14]

Another wonderful mindfulness tool is having an affirmation to say to yourself every day. Similar in theory to mantras (repeated phrases that calm the mind), affirmations are powerful statements meant to boost confidence and deepen the connection to yourself.

Positive and encouraging affirmations are beneficial to both you and your baby, so choose carefully the words you speak, the messages you listen to, and the images you see. You can use one you hear or read from another resource, or even create your own. The only guideline is that your affirmation should resonate powerfully with you. Write down your affirmations, and then say them silently or out loud to yourself throughout the day.

Here are some ideas to get you started:

I am strong and powerful.
I am the leader of my thoughts.
I am safe. All is well.
I love my growing baby and myself.
I nurture my growing baby and myself.
I crave nutritious foods and feed my body and baby well.
I love my powerful and healthy body.

You can talk to your growing baby, as well, several times throughout the day, every day. Gently place both of your hands on your belly as you send him/her/them a loving thought. It can be anything you like, as long as you phrase the message in an affirmative and positive way.

Here are a few examples:

You are wanted.
You are safe.
You are loved.
You are strong and healthy.
I love you.

There is energy in our words. Words can create thoughts and emotions. Words and messages we repeat to ourselves and others on a regular basis create feelings, and those feelings, over time, become beliefs. Choose your words carefully and surround yourself with loved ones and friends who will reinforce your own positive thinking. If you are interested in learning more about the power of affirmations, I recommend looking at the work of Louise Hay.[15] There is also this beautifully written reminder by Mahatma Gandhi[16] about the power of our thoughts and beliefs:

> Your beliefs become your thoughts,
> Your thoughts become your words,
> Your words become your actions,
> Your actions become your habits,
> Your habits become your values,
> Your values become your destiny.

As we turn our attention to the practice of meditation, I encourage you to avoid placing any judgments or values on yourself and your ability to do it. Over the next few pages I will break down for you why meditation is important and how to start your own practice in an accessible way, especially if you are new to it.

Meditation is a way to nourish yourself and also help you see which areas of your life need some extra attention and care. Alas, the idea of sitting down to meditate, even for five minutes, is a daunting one for many people. Some people think that meditation is for a monk sitting on a mountain top, or worry that they are not capable of making their minds go blank. In truth, it is the needless pressure that people put on themselves to "get it right" that makes meditation such a misunderstood practice. The actual purpose of meditation is to find and cultivate the spaces between thoughts. It is simultaneously simple and complex, so let me try to make it more relatable.

Meditation is one of my top three self-care tools. Research is being conducted every day on the benefits of meditation and mindfulness practices for our overall well-being, and more specifically, about its positive effects on the brain and nervous system. Research is also beginning to show that meditation and mindfulness boost positive emotions, counteract the stress response, and decrease depression and anxiety during pregnancy. The most common benefits of a meditation/mindfulness practice span the physical and emotional spheres, and they include: feeling more calm, having more focus, boosting immunity, decreasing anxiety, lowering feelings of depression, and an overall greater sense of well-being. Remember— these are all scientifically proven results.[17]

Meditation is not as esoteric as it might initially seem; in fact, it is actually very logical once we get past the pressure we commonly put on ourselves to instantly get it right. Sitting in quiet reflection brings us closer with our true thoughts and feelings (this is, sometimes, scarier than sitting still). Over time and with dedicated practice, the ability to calm and quiet the mind increases dramatically. Meditation also keeps the negative self-talk at bay because, consciously or not, we all talk to ourselves throughout the entire day. Many of those "discussions" are reflections on things we could have done better. If we are able to replace frenzied, negative thoughts with calm, positive ones, imagine how many of us would be more content in life. Author Steven Campbell says, "The brain is a literal mechanism that accepts what you tell it without argument."[18] As far as I am concerned, we might as well tell it something good!

Meditation also helps us live in the present moment, rather than fretting over the past or worrying about the future. Marianne Williamson gets right to the heart of it when she says, "The present moment, if you think about it, is the only time there is. No matter what time it is, it is always now."[19] The present moment, right now, as you hold this book in your hands, reading these words, is the only thing that is real. The more you cultivate mindfulness and notice where your thoughts go, the easier it will be to harness them and return to the present.

One quick note about where to meditate: It is best to do it seated in a chair or on a cushion/folded blanket on the floor. Many people start their meditation practices by lying in bed right before going to sleep at night. This is a wonderful way to prepare for a more restful sleep, but that is not the purpose of meditation. Therefore, in order to receive all of the benefits of meditation discussed above, it is important to be in an alert state, which is best accomplished in a seated position.

If you would like to add this incredible tool to your self-care routine, begin with five minutes a day a few times (three to five) a week. I encourage you to test out different meditation techniques and find one that works best for you. Are you ready to give it a try? Below are two short and simple meditations that will get you started.

Setting Up for Meditation

- What you will need:
  - A time when you will not be interrupted. Put your phone on mute and close the door.

- A timer. I use the timer on my phone after I have put it in airplane mode.
- A chair or folded blanket or cushion. (A Zafu is a meditation cushion that you can purchase online, if you would like.)
- A shawl or blanket to wrap around your shoulders. (Your body temperature may drop slightly as your body relaxes. It is nice to have something nearby in case you get cold.)

- Sit in a comfortable seated position. If in a chair, place your feet flat on the floor, legs uncrossed. Sit up tall with your chin parallel to the ground.
- Relax your shoulders down and back slightly. Relax all the muscles in your face, especially the point between your eyebrows.
- Place your hands gently in your lap or on your thighs. If you are feeling tired and would like to bring in more energy, place the backs of your hands on your thighs, palms facing up. If you are feeling anxious or energized and would like to be calm and relaxed (before sleep, for example), place your palms down on your thighs to ground your energy. A third hand placement option is laying your right hand, palm up, in your lap, then place your left hand, palm up, resting in your right hand. Touch your thumbs together. This creates a calming effect and helps to relieve agitation and restlessness.
- Relax your belly and the space around your baby.
- Breath in deep, full, and rounded breaths. Never restrict or hold the breath during pregnancy.

- Lower your gaze to the ground; eyelids are heavy or gently closed. Again, allow all the muscles in your face to soften and relax.

- While meditating, allow the corners of your mouth to turn up ever so slightly and the muscles around your eyes to soften. The third eye center, the point between your eyebrows and the seat of your intuition, also relaxes and softens. Relax your tongue inside of your mouth as your top and bottom teeth gently part, releasing your jaw.

Two Simple Styles of Meditation

Repeated Word or Phrase (Mantra Meditation)

This type of meditation supports you to become calmer and more focused. By repeating a word or phrase to yourself, your mind has something to hold on to, keeping other thoughts, worries, planning, or daydreaming at bay. Choose a word or phrase that speaks to you, or try one of the recommendations below. Set your timer for five minutes (or however long you would like) and repeat your chosen "mantra" on each inhalation and exhalation:

* I am calm.
* I breathe in. I breathe out.
* I breathe in peace. I breathe out calm.
* I am safe.
* Om.
* Relax (On inhale, re. . . On exhale, lax).
* Let go (On inhale, let. . . On exhale, go).

Repeat your mantra until you hear your timer sound. If thoughts take over and you find yourself distracted, gently come back to the mantra and continue. Try to withhold judgments on your ability to accomplish this "successfully." There is no right or wrong. There is only practice.

Counting (Counting backwards)

This meditation, like the one above, also focuses on the breath. As you breathe in, you count (to yourself) to a specific number. For example, as you inhale you say to yourself, "ten." As you exhale you say, "nine." Inhale and say, "eight," and so on and so forth. If you get distracted, just come back to the numbers. If you lose your place, simply start again from the top. You will eventually be able to count backwards from 50 or 100. This is an excellent tool to use at night if you are having trouble falling asleep. It will shut off your mind and allow your body to drift off to sleep.

If you would like to learn more about meditation and mindfulness practices, you will find a list of excellent resources at the end of this book.

Pregnancy is a wonderful time to begin a regular meditation practice. Make it your sacred ritual—a special time just for you and your growing baby. Meditation is most effective when practiced regularly, but you will need to determine both the best time of day and best place to practice.

Despite knowing how beneficial a meditation practice can be, it may still be difficult to start. Once you do, though, you will notice the positive effects it is having on your life, and that will hopefully bring you back to the practice time and time again. By implementing these mindfulness and meditation techniques, you will feel calmer, more present, and most importantly, prepared for the arrival of your new baby.

Journal Page

4

yoga and movement

Yoga can create space where there was compression,
can make open what was closed and can make soft our
hard and abrasive edges. The process of pregnancy itself
opens and expands our hearts and our capacity to love.
                                        –Tara Lee, Pregnancy Health Yoga

What type of exercise or movement did you do before becoming
pregnant? Yoga? Daily walking? Swimming? Weights? Pilates?
Exercise can help us to feel more open and alive, and during
pregnancy it becomes even more essential and beneficial for your
well-being and, by extension, your baby. Maintaining a regular
exercise regimen can alleviate swelling in the extremities, improve
heart health and increase blood flow, stabilize your mood, and
strengthen the muscles that assist with labor and delivery.

Pregnancy is not, however, the time to start a vigorous
form of exercise that is new to you. Your body is changing in a
multitude of ways that exert pressure on your internal systems,

and introducing a new high-intensity workout can be more stressful on your body than beneficial. For example, someone who regularly runs marathons might continue her running regimen, adjusting it as her body changes, because she knows how much is too much for her; on the other hand, it would not be beneficial for someone who has never been a runner to suddenly start trying to run a few miles every day because she wants to improve her endurance.

I would, however, encourage bringing new forms of easy movement into your daily routine. I am a certified prenatal yoga teacher, and I practiced yoga several times a week during both of my pregnancies. Yoga supports you in finding balance and union in all aspects of your life. It will improve your physical strength, flexibility, and mental acuity. It also cultivates a strong connection to the present moment. The effects of a yoga practice will relax your body and activate your parasympathetic nervous system (aka "rest and digest" system, and the opposite of the fight-or-flight response).

Prior to getting pregnant the first time, I was a power vinyasa practitioner for several years. (Power Vinyasa Yoga is more active and flowing yoga practice, moving from one posture to the next, connecting the breath to the movements.) I was also a very disciplined person when it came to diet and exercise. I continued to practice power vinyasa in a heated room several times a week after I got pregnant, and I had imposed a strict and rigid self-care routine upon myself. However, as I got further along in my pregnancy, the practice I loved was making me feel more anxious than relaxed.

I had started to worry that the heat and intense postures

(which, despite modifications, still felt advanced for my growing belly) were not beneficial to my baby's health. I had heard many friends confidently announce that they went to hot yoga late into their third trimesters, so I thought that if they could do it, then so could I. After all, this was a practice that had made me feel so good for so many years, so why wouldn't that still be the case?

As I put pressure on myself to "achieve" the same as those around me, I continued to leave classes feeling sad and anxious. It just did not feel right anymore, and during my second trimester, I finally listened to my intuition and tried a prenatal yoga class. It turns out that surrounding myself with other pregnant women while being taught by a knowledgeable prenatal yoga teacher was exactly what I needed.

Yoga is more than a series of postures/poses or stretching. It encompasses breathing techniques, as well as meditation and mindfulness, guided imagery, and relaxation. The main focus of a prenatal yoga is to create a sense of ease for the mother and baby. This is different from other forms of yoga that encourage you to push to your physical edge.

If you normally practice a more intense yoga style, I encourage you to add at least one prenatal yoga class to your schedule. Pay attention not only to how you feel before and after prenatal classes, but also to how you feel before and after a prenatal class versus a more heated and vigorous practice or form of exercise. The differences may surprise you, in that both have diverse effects that are similarly beneficial for you.

If you practice heated vinyasa or go running several miles a day, as many of my friends did during their pregnancies, you may feel completely comfortable with that. Just be sure to listen to signals from your body and your baby, and always make your doctor aware of the activities in which you choose to engage. You may also want to research contraindications of certain yoga postures or exercises. If you normally do other forms of exercise, like Pilates, running, barre, kickboxing, etc., I recommend adding a prenatal yoga class to your routine at least once or twice a week. And, regardless of which form of exercise you choose, always pay close attention to how you feel mentally and physically, before and after each class or session. That awareness will help you structure your exercise regimen to what you need, rather than what you think you have to or should be doing.

Prenatal yoga offers you time to disconnect from the outside world. Leave your cell phone and your to do list outside of the room, along with your shoes and bag. This is an opportunity to have some quiet "me time" and to connect with your growing baby, just the two of you, especially if you have other children at home. This is not to say that you cannot recharge while in cycle class or out for a run; there is, however, a great benefit to slowing down, placing your left hand on your belly and your right hand on your heart, and sending a loving thought to your baby. You will be running around nonstop once your little one arrives, and "me time" will become a rare gift for which we have to create space. Yoga is an opportunity to learn how the quiet times balance the higher energy ones.

The first sixteen weeks of pregnancy are the most delicate. Your body is working extra hard to grow a baby, and in those first few weeks it's setting the stage to accommodate the changes to come. Perhaps women are meant to feel nauseated, lightheaded, and fatigued in the first trimester, because those symptoms, as uncomfortable as they are, may actually prevent us from doing things that have the potential to jeopardize the pregnancy. It is essential, then, that you do not push yourself too hard. If you have a history of miscarriages, it is advised that you not practice yoga at all (even prenatal) or any type of physical exercise during the first sixteen weeks. For others, as long as your doctor gives you the okay, it is generally considered safe.

A regular yoga practice will develop strategies to cope with the discomforts of both pregnancy and birth. So, if you would like to start a prenatal practice, find an experienced and trained yoga instructor who has a prenatal yoga teacher training certification. If there are no prenatal classes near you, then purchasing a DVD to guide you at home is another convenient option; but, if there are studios nearby, then it is worth the effort to go at least once or twice a month. Every studio is unique and they offer different styles, personalities, energies, and ambiance. Find one that is the best fit for you.

A major benefit of taking classes at a studio is getting to practice in a room with a qualified, trained, and knowledgeable instructor. S/he can assist you with your postures and your form to ensure that you are practicing safely. Proper alignment is an important part of yoga, and a teacher can offer instructions and assistance for your specific needs. In the end though, you are your best teacher. You have the final say in how much or how little you do, because you know your body best. If something does not feel right, stop and ask the instructor for a modification or variation.

If your first class does not match up with what you thought it would be, do not give up. You may have to try a few classes/

instructors before you find the combination that fits your needs. Keep in mind, too, that other practitioners are your best resource for suggestions and reviews. Talk to other moms if you are wondering where to go and which instructors to take. Their experiences may actually save you time and money.

Going to a prenatal class offers a wonderful opportunity to meet other moms and find a supportive new community. It is helpful to be able to connect, share, ask questions, and meet other moms-to-be. This is a vital component of self-care. Even if you are shy (like I am) and not always comfortable talking to or meeting new people, it can feel good just to be in the presence of others who are experiencing pregnancy along with you.

There were many times when I went to class and never said a word to anyone; it felt good just to be there. Other times I found myself standing in the lobby chatting with those moms until long after class had ended. I actually met and connected with someone who eventually became a good friend. (Coincidentally, we ended up giving birth within hours of each other on the same day!) If we had not met in the yoga class, we probably would not have connected and developed our friendship.

The three main components of prenatal yoga are: 1) Pranayama—the use of breath and breathing; 2) Asana—the postures and poses; and 3) Savasana—the relaxation that comes at the end. Allow me to briefly explain each of them.

Pranayama (Breath Awareness and Control)

Breathing is a function of the autonomic nervous system, a group of bodily actions that occur without us having to think about doing them (including heart rate, perspiration, digestion, etc.). Pranayama is a powerful breathing technique wherein you focus your attention on your breath to calm both the mind and other systems of the body. Some, but not all, of the benefits of a pranayama practice include: increased oxygen flow to your muscles, improved digestion, reduction in anxiety and depression, lowered blood pressure, and improved immunity. Expectant mothers can use pranayama to help combat fatigue and improve circulation (which can prevent edema, or swelling, in the extremities). As renowned yoga instructor and author Gurmukh says, "As you breathe and as you move, so will your baby throughout his life."[20]

Each practice I highlight in this book is taught by breathing through the nose. This allows the air that enters the body to be moist, warm, and filtered, which is better for the lungs. Before you begin, it is also important to remember that, while pregnant, you do not have much room for deep breathing, because the diaphragm cannot move as much. Be gentle with yourself, but most importantly, do not strain or restrict your breath—allow it to flow continuously.

Below I have outlined three different breathing techniques you can use to calm your mind and relax your body.

Breath Awareness

The balanced breathing practice I am about to discuss is a wonderful place to start if you have never before practiced pranayama. It is the foundation for any advanced breathing practice, and it helps to balance both body and soul. The general idea is to simply make your inhales and exhales the same length.

To begin, find a comfortable seat that allows you to maintain a straight spine for the entire time. Allow your breath to flow naturally at first, noticing it without judgment or effort. After a few moments of observation, you may begin to lengthen the breath. Try to balance the inhalation and exhalation, which can be done by counting as you breathe in, then matching the length/number of the count as you breathe out. If counting the breaths becomes distracting, simply focus on the balance and rhythm between your inhales and exhales. Take five to ten breaths this way, then return to a neutral rhythm and release the control.

Three-Part Breath (Dirga Pranayama)

Sitting comfortably with a straight spine, begin by observing your natural inhalation and exhalation for a few moments. Take in the depth and rhythm without trying to change anything.

To start the Three-Part Breath, breathe in and expand your belly like a balloon. On the exhale, expel all the air out through your nose and allow your belly to release. Repeat this deep belly breathing five times. For the second step of the Three-Part Breath, fill your belly first, then sip in a little more air through your nose and expand your rib cage. Exhale through your nose, allowing your ribs to soften first, and then release your belly. Repeat this sequence five times. For the final component of the three-part breath: breathe in and expand your belly; breathe in more and expand your ribs, then breathe in a little more through your nose to expand your chest and collarbones. Exhale, releasing your chest, then ribs, and finally your belly. Repeat this sequence five times. Once complete, allow your breathing to return to its natural state. Please remember to keep your breath fluid, never restricting or holding your breath.

Alternate Nostril Breathing (Nadi Shodhana Pranayama)

Begin in a comfortable, seated position. If you would like extra support, sit on a folded blanket or cushion. Rest your left hand in your lap, palm facing up. Take a cleansing breath in and gently exhale it out. Place the first and second fingers of your right hand gently on your third eye (the point between your eyebrows). You may instead choose to fold them down into your palm, as shown in drawing below, depending upon which position is more comfortable for you. Close the right nostril with your thumb. Breathe out through the left nostril, then inhale while keeping the right nostril closed, feeling the breath travel up along your spine to the top of your head. Once you have inhaled fully, close the left nostril with the little finger and ring finger and immediately release the thumb to breathe out through the right nostril. Inhale fully through the right nostril, and then close it with your thumb, releasing the ring and pinky fingers on the left nostril and exhale through the left side. Balance the inhalations and exhalations by counting to four each time you breathe in and to four each time you breathe out. Repeat seven times (left inhale, right exhale, right inhale, left exhale = one repetition). Once you have completed seven repetitions, rest both hands gently in your lap, drop your chin slightly, and take a moment to breathe in quiet stillness.

Remember that, while pregnant, you must keep your breath fluid and flowing. Never restrict or hold your breath. If you would like further instruction or to see a visual demonstration of alternate nostril breathing, please go to my website (purenurture. com/free-gifts) for a helpful video.

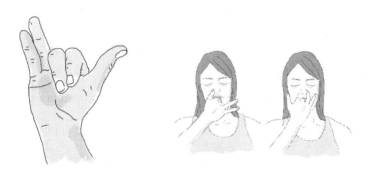

Asana (The Postures/Poses)

Practicing the physical postures of yoga can be both invigorating and relaxing. Prenatal yoga provides an opportunity for you to balance strength and ease (sthira and sukha), just as you will do during labor and delivery. I have highlighted five postures here for you to try and, if possible, practice daily. Each will ultimately help to prepare your body for the physical changes of pregnancy, alleviating any discomfort that may result, as well as preparing for the process of childbirth. If you are new to yoga, please speak with a trained and experienced prenatal yoga teacher (P-RYT) for additional guidance and assistance.

Mountain Pose

Mountain Pose is the foundation for all yoga postures. As your body changes during pregnancy, so will your posture. Your lower back may begin to sway (arch) as the weight of your baby pulls your belly forward. Your shoulders may begin to round as your breasts swell. For these reasons, it is essential to focus on maintaining proper alignment in order to avoid aches and pains down the road.

Begin in bare feet on a flat surface, standing with your feet a little bit wider than hip-width apart. This helps create a more secure and steady base. Lift up all ten toes, spread them wide, then place them gently on the floor again. Sway gently forward and backward, finding your body weight centered between the soles and heels of your feet. Allow your arms to relax by your sides, turning your palms to face forward, thumbs pointing away from your body. Your shoulders relax down and back, without strain, away from your ears. Grow tall through the crown of your head, toward the sky, allowing your spine to lengthen. Your chin is parallel to the ground (imagine you are holding a large orange under your chin). Soften your gaze (drishti) and focus on one point in front of you. Take five to seven deep, relaxed breaths. Release yourself from the pose.

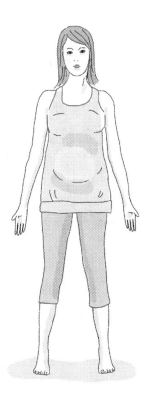

Cat-Cow

This is an all-time favorite of pregnant mamas, because it does so many good things: develops strength and increases energy, helps to relieve tension in the back, and also encourages the baby to move into the ideal birthing position.

To begin, come into a tabletop position on the floor, knees under your hips (hip-width apart) and hands under your shoulders with fingers spread wide like starfish. Gently micro-bend your elbows to bring the weight of your body into your muscles and out of your joints, then turn your elbows slightly inward so that pits of your elbows are facing each other. Your drishti is on the floor, either between or just in front of your hands, allowing your neck to be an extension of your spine. Inhale deeply. As you exhale, lift and round your spine toward the ceiling, gently hugging your baby in. As you're doing this, tuck your chin into your chest (cat pose). Next, inhale as you drop your belly toward the floor, bringing your head up and lifting your chest toward the front of the room. Your spine is now arched, with your tailbone lifting toward the ceiling (cow pose). Repeat five times (one cat and one cow represent one repetition). Let your breath lead you from one posture to the other, ensuring that you never hold or restrict the breath.

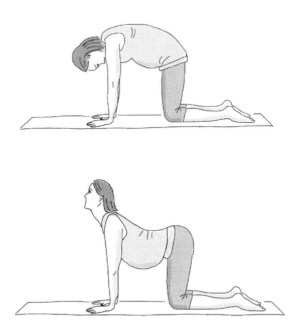

Cobbler's Pose

Sit on a folded blanket. Bring the soles of your feet together and let your knees drop out to the sides. This supports an opening of the hips and a stretching of the inner thighs. If the stretch is too intense, place blocks or another folded blanket under you for added support. Draw your heels toward your groin and place your hands on top of your feet or on your ankles. Hold this seated position for five deep breaths. To come safely out of this pose, place your hands to the outside of your knees and slowly draw them together. Extend your legs out in front of you and shake them out gently. In this position, you can do a seated cat-cow to warm up the spine and stretch the muscles in your back. You can also do hip circles (hip rolls), which help to open the hips and relieve tension and tightness.

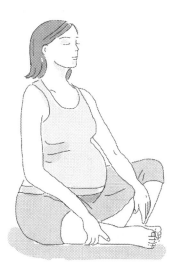

Warrior II

This is a powerful and grounding posture, which provides an excellent opportunity to practice balancing strength with ease. This posture is beneficial because it stretches the hips, groin, and shoulders, and can relieve backaches. It will also help you to build stamina.

To begin, stand with your legs as wide apart as is comfortable.

Pivot your right foot to face away from you, then angle your left foot in forty-five degrees, so that your toes are at a forty-five-degree angle, angled toward your front foot. Lower your hips into a lunge, bringing your right knee to a ninety-degree angle directly over your ankle. Raise your arms until they are parallel to the floor, extending out over your front and back legs. Gaze out over the fingertips of your right hand. Tuck your tailbone slightly down, and hug your baby and belly gently in toward your spine. Breathe deeply for five counts. To come out of the pose, straighten your front leg, pivot your right foot in toward your center, and slowly walk your feet back together. Repeat on the left side.

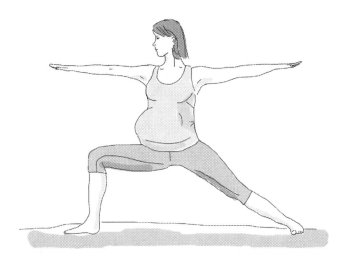

Tree Pose

All balancing postures seek to create harmony between the

two sides of the body. This pose balances both sides of the brain, as well as the systems of the body. It also helps pregnant women find a new center of gravity as their bellies expand and their equilibrium is altered.

Begin standing in Mountain Pose (as described above). Ground down through your left foot, creating a strong, stable base. Place the sole of your right foot against the inside of the standing ankle, calf, or inner thigh (avoid placing your foot on your knee joint). Join your hands together in front of your heart center, pressing your palms together. Set your drishti to one unmoving spot in front of you, and take five calm, focused breaths. It is okay if you wobble out. Simply come back to the posture and try again. Repeat on the other side.

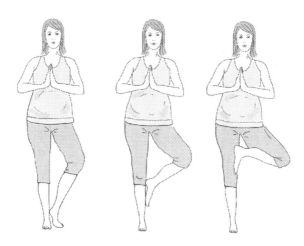

Savasana (Final Relaxation)

At the end of most yoga classes or practices, everyone rests in final relaxation, or Savasana. Savasana means "corpse pose" in Sanskrit, the intention being complete and total stillness so that the body may become calm and the mind may focus more clearly. It allows for a time when the energy generated by a physical practice can be absorbed by the body. This will balance the nervous system, which encourages healing and relaxation.

Since it is advised that women not lay on their backs after the first trimester, I recommend that you lay on your left side with a bolster or a firm pillow supporting the top leg and a folded blanket under the head. This position will allow the spine and hips to remain in alignment and prevent pressure on the vagus nerve. It also allows for deep relaxation.

Please see the Resources section at the end of the book for more information related to prenatal yoga, including books and videos.

Prenatal Yoga Benefits:

- Increases muscle strength
- Creates a sense of community
- Calms nervous system
- Brings more oxygen into the body
- Improves circulation
- Reduces swelling and varicose veins
- Increases perineal strength (helps with pre- and post-partum pelvic floor control)
- Normalizes blood pressure
- It feels good!

Journal Page

Here is a list of questions to ask yourself before and after each session/practice/class to help you determine what feels best for you and your baby:

1. Do I feel invigorated or exhausted afterwards?
2. Do I feel stronger or weaker?
3. Do I feel at ease or anxious?

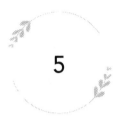

5

more ways to nurture yourself

Let us make pregnancy an occasion when
we appreciate our female bodies.
—Merete Leonhardt-Lupa, A Mother is Born

There are many self-care activities and practices that will improve your health and the health of your baby, if applied throughout your pregnancy. I have made a list of suggestions for activities you can do alone as well as therapies you may want to try by finding a practitioner in your area.

Rest and Sleep

The difference between "sleep" and "rest" may seem nuanced, but it is actually quite defined. Sleep is a period of unconsciousness and cessation of voluntary movement in which your body recovers from the day, while rest is a conscious pause in your activities in order to regain strength or energy. The distinction matters because pregnancy requires you to not only sleep more but also take time to rest and restore.

It is important to increase the amount of time you sleep so that your body may adapt to the physical changes happening within. Listen to your body's need for sleep. If you feel tired and are able, take a nap, and later, try your best to get a good night's sleep.

Slowing down is equally essential. I know that this will be difficult if you are the type of person who hates to stop or dislikes feeling unproductive, but you need to start adjusting your definition of "getting things done." The truth is that it boils down to perspective—while you may not be physically moving and accomplishing things, internally you are very active. Another important point is to remember that you are not fully resting if you are on your phone, watching TV, or using your computer, so avoid screen time for between one and two hours before you go to bed.

Journal Writing

It is important to release thoughts and feelings (good or bad) that may weigh you down in any way. Some people like to talk to friends or family, but many people experience journaling as a cathartic exercise in self-exploration. As author Steven Levine said, "When the mind is clear, you can see all the way to the heart."[21] Journaling helps you tap into the deeper knowledge of yourself that exists beyond intellect and ego because, when you let go of the things that normally clog your mind, you get to know yourself better. This ultimately enables you to determine what you truly want or need. True self-care can only happen when you see yourself clearly.

If traditional journaling doesn't feel right for you, another idea is to create a Gratitude Journal. Keep a list of things, big and small, for which you feel grateful. You can also write what you love or enjoy about being pregnant. Struggle with anxiety or worrying thoughts, especially at night? Writing down a list of five or more reasons to be thankful for what you have can be a wonderful addition to your bedtime routine. Positivity is key, however it is not always easy to access. If you sometimes have difficulty identifying the better parts of a hard day, here are some ideas to get you started that other mamas have used:

I loved…

- Watching my belly grow.
- Feeling my baby move and kick.
- Fostering a connection with him before birth.
- How considerate and kind strangers were with me.

You may find yourself expressing worries or concerns while journaling, but I recommend being mindful of putting too much negativity on paper all at once. If you use your journal to vent, to recap the happenings of your day, or to sort out your ideas and thoughts about things to come, consider concluding your entry with a positive thought so as to bring balance to your day. This will allow your mind and emotions to slow down and even themselves out.

Massage

When you're pregnant and carrying the physical weight of

your baby, as well as the responsibilities of becoming a parent, it is not selfish to go the extra mile to make sure you take care of yourself. Too often the things that will make us feel better are considered an "indulgence," and we may shy away from them, because we do not want people to think that we are self-centered. I take the opposite stance and choose to believe that treating yourself well is a necessity, and I encourage you to embrace any opportunity to give yourself a little more attention. You actually need that extra care in order to keep yourself happy and calm during these nine months (and beyond).

Bodywork, such as massage, is often viewed as a luxury for someone who has time and money, but the truth is that it plays a vital role in maintaining a healthy and balanced body. Massage is beneficial for several reasons. It clears the body of tension, recharges physical energy, and frees our minds from preoccupying thoughts, among others. I recommend booking regular massages so that you have them on the calendar, and if you start to tell yourself that you are "too busy" with other things to make an appointment, try instead to be busy taking care of you.

If you feel disinclined to pay for bodywork yourself, ask for a massage as a birthday gift, holiday gift, or as a baby shower present. If coworkers ask what you need for the baby, tell them you need a massage. People will be delighted to give you something you really love and need. If paying for a massage is outside of your budget, you can do a self massage, especially on your feet, or request regular massages from your spouse, partner, or a good friend.

Some of the benefits of massage are that it:

- Improves quality of sleep
- Relieves and reduces back pain
- Improves and increases circulation
- Reduces stress and anxiety
- Reduces muscle tension, tightness, and headaches

Conserving Your Energy

Protecting your energy is never more important than when you are pregnant. Gurmukh says, "Putting too many demands on yourself actually contracts your body instead of creating space."[22] Creating space is essential to good health and well-being because contraction and constriction lead to pain, discomfort, and illness, both emotionally and physically.

We are all so very busy today, something I like to call "busy-itis." "Sorry I haven't called, I've just been so busy," we tell our friends and family. It has become a very socially acceptable response. We wear busy-ness as a badge of honor, as if it means that we are important or needed or successful.

How can we become less busy? How can we slow down? For starters, we can say "no" more often, and without guilt. That last part is key, because agreeing to things you do not want to do can sap your energy very quickly. Take a moment to consider how you feel when making a decision about whether or not to attend a holiday party or other social event. Are you excited to see everyone? Do you feel energized by the idea of attending, or do you feel overwhelmed and exhausted by the idea of it? Obligations aside, if you are not looking forward to a particular event or get together, honor your feelings and say, "No, thank you," in a very polite and graceful way. Then drop any guilt you might feel about saying no. Your number one priority during pregnancy is nourishing and nurturing your growing baby, and there is only so much energy to go around, so conserve it where you can. This is the core tenet of self-care: putting your baby and yourself first.

Everything is made of energy. Now, I don't want to get too esoteric on you or discuss quantum physics, but it is worth mentioning that there is growing evidence of how energy flows and how it affects our health. The book *E2, E-Squared*, by Pam Grout, describes experiments you can do to prove to yourself the existence of your own energy field.[23] Having done the experiments myself, I can tell you that it is fascinating to see how energy moves. One involves bending wire coat hangers to use as your own divining rods. I was blown away by the immediate effect my thoughts had on the movement of the wire hangers. It felt like they were possessed! I called my husband into the room so that we could both try it.

After we each did our own experiment, we took it a step further. We played "lie detector test." We asked each other silly questions to see which direction the wires would point. (To set it up, you straighten out two wire coat hangers so that they stick out in front of you, and then hold them close to your body while you ask questions or conjure thoughts.) The two wires moving together represented closed energy (no); the two wires moving apart, represented open energy (yes).

My hubby asked me, "Do you want to have sex tonight?" (In my defense, it was 11:30 p.m. on a Tuesday night, and I was exhausted.) Well, with all my other questions, for a "no" or "contraction" the hangers would meet and tap together. For a "yes" they spread wide apart. For this specific question, as soon as he finished asking, the wire hangers closed quickly together, tapping at the center, and they didn't stop there. They crossed all the way, forming an X across my body, as if they were yelling "Hell NO!!" We couldn't stop laughing at that visual.

Well, it was all fun and games until my clever husband mentioned Adam Levine of Maroon 5 in his next question. Believe me when I tell you that those wires opened up so quickly! I threw them down on the floor and yelled, "No! No incriminating questions!" Again, we shared a good laugh. (Luckily my husband isn't the jealous type, not to mention that the odds of Adam Levine coming over to visit are pretty slim.)

The point of this story is not about my sex life or dreams about Adam Levine, but to help you get an idea of how powerful your thoughts are, and how strongly they can affect your life. Everything is energy, and it is up to you to protect yours.

Say Yes to What is Best and No to the Rest

Saying "no" in order to honor time and your needs is the wisest thing you can do for you and your baby. If you want to stay home with your hubby, say no to the girls. If you feel an afternoon with your sister is exactly what you need, tell your husband he is on his own for the day. Setting boundaries can be a great way to protect your energy. You only have so much time and energy to go around, especially when pregnant. Two key areas I'd like to highlight are boundaries in the context of your relationships with others and in relation to external stimuli, such as television programs, movies, news broadcasts, etc.

You may have heard this next suggestion before, that is to only surround yourself with others who uplift, inspire and support you. Anyone that is negative or draining may do just that: drain you and bring you down. After meeting with a friend or getting off the phone, ask yourself how you feel. Do you feel full or do you feel drained? Surround yourself more often with others that leave you feeling better.

In regards to the media you consume, even though you cognitively understand the events are on a flat screen, and many times the people are just portraying characters in a made-up plot, your physical body will release stress hormones like cortisol and your muscles will tense as though it is really happening to you personally. Some women will be more affected by external stimuli than others. Some of you may love to watch horror films, while others, like me, are affected for days afterward. Moreover, during your pregnancy, you may even find that your reactions are different; maybe you will find that things that normally wouldn't bother you start to get under your skin. When you are pregnant, the emotions you feel can transfer to the baby. In his book, *The Biology of Belief*, author Bruce Lipton dedicates an entire chapter to conscious parenting, where he shares information and research regarding how the fetus is directly impacted by the mother's stress levels, thoughts, and more.[24] You know yourself best, and I only offer this as an idea to ponder and consider. If you are easily impacted by negative stimuli, you may want to consider only watching, reading, and listening to that which inspires you, makes you laugh, or brings you comfort.

Journal Page

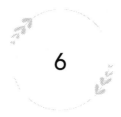

6

your pregnancy tribe

It takes a village to raise a child.

—African proverb

Throughout the world, especially in less economically developed countries, women join forces to help a mother grow, deliver, and raise her child(ren). On the other hand, Western societies typically view pregnancy as an individual's, rather than a community's, responsibility. It is, therefore, not uncommon for pregnant women in our society to feel isolated and alone. Tony Robbins, motivational speaker and author, talks about the six core human needs, which include Connection and Love.[25] Feeling connected to something or someone is essential to our overall well-being; I believe that when we are pregnant, the desire for closeness and support increases and becomes even more important than usual. I even tend to imagine that there are missing words implied in the quotation above, amending it to "it takes a village to raise a child, starting from conception."

Part of your self-care during pregnancy and as a mother is to communicate your needs. We will never get what we want if we do not tell people about it. I was raised to believe that if someone truly loves me, then I should never have to express what I need because s/he should automatically know what to do and when. In real life, though, people are not mind-readers. Reconciling what I was told with the reality of human behavior is, to this day, something I work on in my relationships. In order to avoid feelings of resentment and passive-aggressive behaviors, it is vital to share your thoughts and emotions with those around you. By expressing yourself in a kind and respectful way, not only will you find support where you and your baby need it most, your loved ones will also feel more capable of helping you through this life-changing time.

Pregnancy is a significant transition in a woman's life. It is not, however, given the depth of attention that other transitions, such as marriage, motherhood, and divorce, are afforded. Pregnancy affects a woman on every level—physically, psychologically, and spiritually: it can lead a woman to love her body more than ever, or turn her against it because of the changes it goes through; it can elevate her spirits or bring her down, depending on how it alters her hormones; it also has the potential to build deeper connections to others, or to isolate due to its otherness.

No one can deny that social media and texting has brought together those who were far apart. Thanks to Facebook, Twitter, Instagram, etc., you now know what the girl who sat next to you in second grade had for dinner last night. It has also, conversely, decreased the need for face-to-face interaction. Even phone calls have been replaced with texting. Yes, you still know how things are going with your BFF because you text every day, but do you remember the sound of her voice or how comforting it is to hear her laugh? The loss of such sensory reminders can increase feelings of isolation for someone who is already struggling with loneliness, especially during pregnancy.

So what is the solution? *Gasp* Connect with people face-to-face. Think about who around you provides support, love, guidance, and care. Seek out those people and create your community. Even if you rarely ask for or accept help from others, allow them to support you. This is not the time to emulate Wonder Woman, multitasking and working up to the very last possible minute before giving birth. You do not have to travel through these nine months alone, so allow others to support you.

Take a few minutes to think of the names of people and groups in your life who help you feel cared for and supported. This can include friends, family, coworkers, neighbors, teachers, groups, classes, organizations, therapists, etc. How do you feel about your tribe? Can you depend on these people when you need some extra support? If so, do not wait on them to call you—just go ahead and reach out. Instead of taking it personally if a friend is not calling, simply pick up the phone and call him/her yourself. Both you and your friend will be happy you did.

Activating the "Buddy System" or designating an accountability partner is a good way to stay invested in your self-care. Partner up with someone you care about and trust (pregnant or not) and become "Self-Care Accountability Partners." You can create an "accountability schedule" that meets both of your needs. You can set up a call once a week or every other week for twenty minutes to an hour and even add an email/text exchange in between your calls just to say a quick hello. It is up to you and your partner to figure out what works best.

Your Professional Team

Your team of professionals is just as important as your family and friends. It may include one or more of the following specialists: OB, Midwife, Doula, Massage Therapist, Mental Health Therapist, Life Coach, Prenatal Yoga Teacher, and/or Prenatal Health Coach. It is important to ask yourself: How do they talk to you? Are they respectful of your wishes and concerns? Do they communicate with fear-based information, or are they positive and affirmative? Do they spend quality time with you?

If you answer "no" to those questions, or if for any reason you do not feel 100% comfortable with the care you are receiving, do not hesitate to shop around for a new practitioner. It is important to know that it is never too late to switch doctors or other health care services. Whether you have been with your OB for years and then decide that you are not happy with him/her, or you feel certain you want a doula at your birth but your OB is opposed to the idea, you are within your rights to find someone who meets all, or most, of your needs. Do not compromise on the things about which you feel the strongest. You will know what they are, and you have the right to find someone who (within reason) supports your choices.

Silence Your Inner Critic

Pregnancy is a time full of self-evaluation and self-criticism.

The Internet has granted us access to a plethora of information on pregnancy and parenting: medicated vs. natural births; to vaccinate or not; yes or no to caffeine during pregnancy; breast milk vs. formula. The list goes on. The effects of this heightened awareness are an increase in value-laden judgments about what kind of parent you will be/already are.

The best defense against this kind of feedback is to let go of the judgments and comments from others. Easier said than done, I know, but just like meditation, this is a practice. There are a lot of opinionated people out there eager to tell everyone that they know best. Instead of stressing about their opinions, disconnect from them altogether. In fact, you do NOT have to listen to anyone who shares comments about your choices, your body, or their pregnancy stories. If what you hear is anything but positive, loving, affirmative, and kind, then tune it out. Make it very clear what you will and will not tolerate, because you have every right to teach others how to treat you. For example, if someone starts sharing her birth story, you have every right to stop her and ask if she had a positive experience. If she says no, feel free to tell her that you would like to hear about her experience—AFTER you give birth.

As you progress through your forty or so weeks, your wants and needs may change. Empower yourself to practice self-care by making the changes necessary to feel your best. I emphasize this point because nine-plus months of pregnancy are not all sugar plums and daffodils. There is plenty of unpleasantness. I do not know of one woman who had a seamless and smooth pregnancy, although some will say they did. The first time someone asked me about my pregnancy, I said, "I loved it. It was amazing. I loved being pregnant!" Less than a second later, my husband cleared his throat loudly and said, "Are you sure about that? That's not how I remember it." He was right. And no, I was not lying. I just truly remembered it that way. There is supposedly a hormone that, over time, allows women to feel less affected by the difficulties of pregnancy and childbirth. Maybe that is how Mother Nature ensures we continue on?

Pregnancy is a miracle. It is an amazing and beautiful experience. It is also, at times, exhausting and uncomfortable, so do not worry when you feel less than excited about being pregnant. That is normal, and if you have the people you need around you, then you can support each other along the way.

Journal Page

7

pulling it all together

The health of every family begins with the mother. She
is the tree from which the healthy fruit must come.
— Juliette de Bairacli Levy, Nature's Children

Every journey comes with its trying moments, and pregnancy is no different. People who care deeply about you (or perhaps whom you have never even met before) will give you their advice, regardless of whether or not you want to hear it: opinions about what you should and should not do, can and cannot do, etc. They will eagerly share their experiences with you, because we moms (yes, even me) LOVE to do that. More often than not we are approaching you with the best intentions to help and share our memories, but you, the one with the baby in your belly right now, may or may not want to hear from us. And then there is the Internet. The things people share and criticize and judge from the protection of their computer screens, not to mention all of the medical articles that provide conflicting information... oh, boy.

As a new mom, all of this information at your fingertips can be incredibly overwhelming, which is why the final chapter of this book is designed to empower you to do what feels best for YOU.

There is no such thing as doing your pregnancy "right," at least not in a one-size-fits-all way. Women will tell you, "Oh, I didn't drink one drop of coffee or one drop of alcohol. It's so bad for the baby!" or "Oh, I had a coffee every day, it is totally ok. My child is healthy as a horse!" or "A little wine here and there won't hurt anything." You may hear something along the lines of, "Don't step foot in a sushi restaurant!" to which someone else will inevitably say, "I ate cooked sushi throughout my pregnancy." You may feel a push-pull of advice, or marvel at the contradictions in people's personal stories.

It is easy to hold yourself up to imaginary standards or self-imposed judgments and rules. The truth is, though, that in partnership with a doctor or midwife you trust, the only person who knows what is right for you, is you. For just this moment in time, let go of all that and consider that you are doing the very best you can. Listen to your body. Listen to what your intuition is telling you. Listen closely to that small, quiet voice that resides deep inside your gut. That voice will support your self-care if you allow it to guide you in creating and maintaining your physical and spiritual balance.

All of this is to say that your best friends' suggestions—and even this book—are a supplement to what you are instinctually doing to support your growing baby. In reality, you take in what feels best for you and your baby and leave behind what does not fit. When people spontaneously tell you how they think you should be handling your pregnancy, patiently and respectfully listen to their well-intentioned comments, and then go do whatever you know to be right for you and your baby.

Gurmukh said, "Everything you do for yourself you are doing for the soul within you, to relax, to eat well, to meditate, to be with good friends, to read wonderful books, your baby is taking all of it in like a sponge."[26] Bringing a baby into the world is a big responsibility, so if you approach it from a place of love, knowing that all you can do is try your best, you will instinctually do what needs to be done.

Since different self-care activities will work better for some than others, I asked a few friends and clients to share about their pregnancy journey and their favorite self-care practices. In their own words:

Jenn: I loved the "protected state" of pregnancy. I felt fantastic and had so much more energy than I did in everyday life. Sex, hands down, was the best! I loved pregnant sex. Watching my body change and grow was incredible. For the first time in a long time, I felt comfortable in my own skin. I loved my big belly, and I felt like a goddess most of the time. When I wasn't feeling so great my biggest complaints were my lower back and heartburn and that feeling that "my vagina is falling out!" To help with these issues and just to continue feeling my best while pregnant, I would get chiropractic adjustments, go swimming, and get prenatal massages. Yoga really helped maintain my physical and mental happiness. Warm baths were extremely soothing as well.

Finally, I would recommend everyone splurge on a few pieces of maternity clothing that make you feel fantastic!

Gabrielle: I loved feeling my babies move and kick. I felt like I was living a cool science experiment. I also really enjoyed fostering a special bond with my babies before they were born. No one else had that connection with them that I had, and I felt they were familiar to me on the day they were born. It was amazing how friendly strangers were to me. They would hold the door, warned me to stay away if they were sick, and extend congratulations and pleasantries. My self-care practices during pregnancy were to take brisk walks, attend yoga classes, go swimming, eat healthy foods, or take a warm bath. Whenever I was feeling sick or exhausted, one of these things usually helped me to feel better.

Vivienne: I was nauseated all the way to my fifth month of pregnancy. To help with the nausea, I ate every two hours. The key was to never let myself get hungry. Bananas were my go-to snack, and they helped to ease the nausea. As the baby grew, she was pushing on my stomach, so I was only able to eat small amounts, so eating every two hours made sense for me. One aspect of pregnancy that I felt was lacking was related to the actual birth. I would have liked to have been more prepared mentally and emotionally. I'm very grateful I had a Doula during my labor and delivery. It made the experience in the hospital much more relaxing and intimate.

April: The first three months of my pregnancy I had morning sickness that lasted all day and night. When I became pregnant I wanted to eat well, but when I couldn't keep down vegetables or fruits, the only thing I found to help was a chicken sandwich (and not the healthy kind). It was, unfortunately, my go-to for the first three months. It was such a staple my husband didn't need to ask what was for dinner... on his way home from work he knew he better grab me this sandwich or else. I quickly learned that I had to adjust to what my body was feeling, and eventually one of my cravings was vegetables with ranch. I also found that long walks soothed me. I loved getting prenatal massages, and taking a warm bath, sometimes several a day, helped too. My body, especially my lower back, was a huge problem area during pregnancy. If I could do it over again, I would try prenatal yoga. I do not do yoga on a regular basis, so the fear of looking like I didn't fit in stopped me from going. I wish now that I wouldn't have let this stop me.

Dianne: Other than being a little nauseous during the first couple months, my pregnancy was not marked with too many ailments or complaints. The two issues I dealt with most were back pain and feeling very tired. To help with this I would take walks outside every day. Breathing in fresh air and being outside moving my body helped to relieve the fatigue. The prenatal yoga and Pilates DVDs I had helped me to feel stronger and more energetic too. I would alternate them and use them several times a week. I always felt like I needed to be doing something to get things ready before the baby arrived. I almost felt like I was being lazy if I wanted to sleep all day. One thing I wish is that I had someone to tell me that it's ok to be tired and rest. One time I booked myself a spa day and got pampered. It was awesome!

In closing, I want to encourage you to make yourself your priority as you prepare for your baby's arrival. Nothing will be perfect, no one does everything right every minute of every day, and you will find yourself making different decisions than other moms around you. But if you practice self-care in a way that feels true to you and carry your self-care tips and tools with you into your days as a new mom, you will find a sense of peace amongst the chaos of life.

Wishing you and your little one(s) much love, compassion, health, nurturance, and peace,

Kristy

May the long time sun shine upon you. All love surround you. And the pure light within you, Guide your way on.

—Mike Heron, A Kundalini Farewell Blessing.

Bonus Chapter

recipes!

All recipes created by Elise Museles of Kale & Chocolate

I am a firm believer that what you put in your body is a huge component of being a self-care mama. Nothing makes you feel as good from the inside out the way colorful and nutrient-filled food does! Healthy eating isn't about measuring, weighing, or following a strict meal plan. It means enjoying whole, real food.

We stay away from the word "diet" because this is a lifestyle. The more you eat "real food," the better you will feel. When you fill your plate with deeply pigmented fruits & veggies, grains, legumes, healthy fats, and clean proteins, the less room you will have for the not-so-good-for-you foods.

I am delighted to team up with my good friend, an eating psychology & health coach, Elise Museles. Elise is a writer, speaker, recipe developer, and the voice behind the insightful blog Kale & Chocolate. She is also the author of the book, *Whole Food Energy* (Barron's Educational Series, January 2016).

I knew that I had to have Elise create some nutrient-dense recipes especially for you. Use these mini-meals and light bites to keep your blood sugar even throughout the day, curb cravings, and nip nausea in the bud. Soon enough, you can come up with your own combinations of nutritious (and delicious!) pregnancy superfoods, too!

SMOOTHIES

Smoothies are an excellent way to pack in a lot of pregnancy superfoods. In just a few minutes, you can create a nutrient-dense meal or snack tailored to your specific tastes or needs. Begin with these recipes, and then start filling your blender with your own colorful creations. Once you get blending, there's no turning back!

Strawberry Shortcake Smoothie

Although this smoothie may look basic upon first glance, it is anything but basic. Loaded with antioxidants, a mega-dose of vitamin C, plus lots of flavor, one serving includes a delicious boost of nutrients reminiscent of a tasty dessert. This is equally satisfying first thing in the morning to kick-start a busy day as it is as a mid-afternoon pick-me-up that will keep blood sugar even and steady!

*Serves 1–2

Ingredients
1 cup plant-based milk (almond, cashew, or coconut milk work well)

1–2 tablespoons raw cashews

1 ¼ cups frozen strawberries

½ large banana, sliced & frozen

½ teaspoon vanilla

1 teaspoon lemon zest (don't skip this!)

Pinch of sea salt

Method

Blend the cashews and the plant-based milk in a high-speed blender until smooth. Add in remaining ingredients and blend until a creamy consistency is reached. Use additional nut milk if necessary for a thinner consistency. Sip, savor, and enjoy!

Get Your Green On Smoothie

For a tasty way to flood your body with plant-based nutrients, load your blender up with heaps of greens. While this smoothie is filled with lots of veggies, it is also hydrating, good for digestion (hello pineapple and ginger!), and refreshing!

*Serves 1–2

Ingredients

1 cup coconut water

1 handful kale, stalks removed

1 handful spinach

2 celery stalks

2 Romaine leaves

½ inch piece of fresh ginger, peeled

2 tablespoons parsley

2 tablespoons lime juice (can use lemon juice)

pinch of sea salt

1 cup frozen pineapple

½ large ripe pear (provides creaminess)

Method

Blend the coconut water, kale, and spinach together until smooth. Add in the remaining ingredients and blend until well-combined. Adjust desired consistency by adding more or less of the coconut water. Enjoy!

SMOOTHIE BOWLS

(See the Topping Chart for more superfood inspiration to add to your bowl.)

For a smoothie that feels like a meal, whip up an extra-creamy smoothie bowl that tastes like soft serve ice cream. Filled with the same nutritious ingredients as a classic smoothie, but with a thicker consistency and fun toppings that provide a nutritional boost that a busy mama or mama-to-be could use!

Blueberry Baby Bliss

Filled with lots of nutrient-dense ingredients, this beautiful blueberry smoothie recipe is sure to help you start your day out on the right note. With blueberries, almonds, spinach, and avocados all in one place, your body will be thanking you all morning long. Don't forget to sprinkle on some toppings for an extra nutritional boost.

*Serves 1–2

Ingredients

6 ounces almond milk (use coconut milk for a nut-free version)

1 cup frozen blueberries (or any berry combination works)

2 handfuls spinach

¼–½ avocado

½ teaspoon vanilla

1–2 pitted Medjool dates or ½ banana, sliced & frozen

Pinch of sea salt

Optional: 2 tablespoons vanilla plant-based protein powder

Note: for a sweeter smoothie, use the whole frozen banana.

Method

Place almond milk and spinach in a high-speed blender and puree until smooth. Blend in protein powder (optional). Add remaining ingredients and blend until desired consistency is reached. This is a thick smoothie. Add a drop more almond milk, if necessary. Top with any combination of fresh fruit, seeds, nuts, superfoods, or granola. Get creative. Whip out a spoon and dig in!

It's Easy Being Green

Loaded with just as many greens as the more traditional green smoothies, the green smoothie bowl is the perfect way to add in a nutritional punch to your day. Start with this base and then vary the greens depending on tastes and availability. The variety of toppings creates endless possibilities to cover your body's varying (and changing!) needs.

*Serves 1

Ingredients

6 ounces plant-based milk

2 cups leafy greens, loosely packed (spinach, kale, Swiss chard, or any combo)

¼ avocado

1 banana, sliced & frozen

Pinch of sea salt

Optional flavorings: vanilla, cinnamon, lemon zest, ginger, or mint

Method

Blend the greens and plant-based milk. Add in remaining ingredients and blend until smooth. Adjust to desired consistency with additional plant-based milk, if necessary. Put in a bowl and cover with toppings of choice. Get creative and have fun!

TOPPING INSPIRATION (For Smoothie Bowls)

Topping:	What Makes It Great: (The Top 3 Nutrients*)
Cacao nibs	Antioxidants, Fiber. and Magnesium
Shredded coconut	Protein, Fiber, Iron, and Zinc
Goji berries	Vitamin C, B2, and Potassium
Mulberries	Resveratrol, Vitamin C, and Iron
Fresh fruit (mangos, kiwi, berries, chopped figs, sliced bananas, peaches, pomegranate seeds)	Extremely high in antioxidants and a wide variety of vitamins and minerals.

Hemp seeds	Protein, Omegas 3, 6, and 9, and all 9 Essential Amino Acids
Chia seeds	Fiber, Protein, and Antioxidants
Pumpkin seeds	Magnesium, Protein, and Zinc
Sunflower seeds	Copper, Manganese, and Calcium
Nuts (cashews, sliced almonds, crushed walnuts, pecans, Macadamia nuts) Granola	Omegas 3, 6, and 9, Protein, and B Vitamins (including folate)
Fresh mint leaves	Manganese, Copper, and Vitamin C
Drizzles of nut or seed butter	Omegas 3, 6, and 9, Protein, and B Vitamins (including folate)

*The nutritional value and benefits of each superfood are too many to list here. If you'd like to learn more, please consult with trusted sources.

BABY FRITTATAS

All the same nutrients and protein in a regular-sized frittata but made in handy muffin cups for an easy individual, grab and go option. Use this recipe as a springboard to create your own variations, mixing seasonal veggies or whatever your body may be craving (or needing!). Make a tray ahead of time and then store it in the refrigerator for up to two days or in the freezer for up to one month. Simply pull one out to reheat whenever you need a quick protein-packed bite.

*Serves 6

Ingredients
1 tablespoon olive oil, plus more for greasing the muffin tray
¼ cup red bell peppers, diced and seeds removed
½ cup spinach, thinly sliced
½ cup onion, diced
¼ cup mushrooms, chopped in small pieces
½ teaspoon salt
¼ teaspoon ground pepper
12 large eggs (use hormone-free, if possible)
splash of water (or use unsweetened plant-based milk or milk)
Sprinkling of shredded cheese of choice (optional)

Method
Preheat the oven to 350 degrees and lightly oil the muffin tray.

In a large pan, heat the olive oil and then add the prepared red peppers, spinach, onion, and mushrooms. Sauté on medium-high heat for 3–4 minutes until the vegetables begin to soften. Set aside. Whisk the eggs in a medium-large mixing bowl and add a splash of water. Season with salt & pepper. Fold in the sautéed vegetables and mix well. Pour the egg mixture into the muffin pans until about three-quarters full. Sprinkle the cheese on top, if using. Bake for about 22–25 minutes, removing from the oven once the top is golden brown and the eggs are set in the middle. Enjoy!

CHIA SEED PUDDING

This small seed produces big benefits. Aside from being a nutritional powerhouse filled with an easily digestible form of protein that is a rich source of iron, magnesium, calcium, and phosphorous, chia seeds have also been touted to help with achy joints. Try this delicious and omega-rich chia seed pudding for breakfast, snack or dessert. It can even be layered with a smoothie to create a chia seed parfait!

*Serves 4

Ingredients
½ cup chia seeds
2 cups plant-based milk (almond, hemp, coconut)
3 tablespoons coconut nectar or pure maple syrup
½ teaspoon pure vanilla extract or vanilla powder
Pinch of sea salt

Pregnancy Superfood Add-ins

Cinnamon
Cardamom
Mesquite
Lemon zest (so good!)
Matcha green tea powder
Raw cacao or unsweetened cocoa powder

Note: To make a smaller batch, simply cut the recipe in half.

Method

Pour all ingredients into a bowl. Stir until well combined. Allow to sit for 30 minutes whisking every 10 minutes until mixture thickens. Place in the refrigerator and store for several hours or overnight. Check for desired thickness and flavor. Adjust if needed. When ready to serve, spoon the pudding into bowls (or store in mason jars) and top with fresh berries. Enjoy! Keeps in the refrigerator for up to 4 days.

HEMP SEED HUMMUS

While hummus in and of itself is an excellent (and tasty!) way to load up on fiber and plant-based protein, the hemp seeds add a healthy dose of omega-rich fatty acids. For a portable option, fill the bottom of a Mason jar with a serving of hummus and then stick in some sliced veggies. Seal the lid and voila—hummus to go as you run out the door.

*Serves 6

Ingredients

1 ½ cups garbanzo beans (one BPA-free 15-ounce can)
2 tablespoons lemon juice
1 garlic clove
¼ cup tahini
3 tablespoons hemp seeds
½ teaspoon cumin
1 teaspoon lemon zest
½ teaspoon sea salt (or to taste)
2–4 tablespoons water

Top with chopped Italian flat leaf parsley, hemps seeds, paprika, and a drizzle of olive oil

Method

Rinse and drain the garbanzo beans. Place the garbanzo beans, lemon juice, garlic, and tahini in the food processor and process until combined. Add in the cumin, lemon zest, hemp seeds, and salt and process. With the motor running, slowly drizzle in water until the desired consistency is reached. Process until completely smooth and creamy, scraping down the sides of the container if necessary. Adjust seasonings to taste.

Transfer to a bowl and serve with chopped Italian flat leaf parsley, a sprinkle of hemp seeds, paprika, and a drizzle of olive oil.

Note: if the hummus thickens in the refrigerator, add a drop of water to reconstitute before serving.

GUAC-KALE-MAMA

Guac-Kale-Mama brings guacamole to a whole new nutrient-dense level. How can you go wrong when you mix kale with avocado? Make sure to soften the kale by massaging it first with a drop of olive oil so that it blends well with the creamy avocado. Mash all the ingredients just like traditional guacamole, then give it some extra green love with the addition of thinly sliced kale!

*Serves 6

Ingredients
2–3 avocados

1 lime, juiced

¼ cup red onion, chopped

½ clove garlic, chopped

½–1 jalapeño pepper, chopped

2 tablespoons cilantro, chopped

¼ teaspoon cumin

½ teaspoon sea salt (plus more to taste)

4 large kale leaves, stalk removed

Method

Mix and mash ingredients together (except kale) in a bowl to desired consistency. Massage kale (stalks removed) with a drop of olive oil to soften. Next, thinly slice by hand or process in a food processor. (Make sure not to over-process if using a food processor.) Once sliced, add the kale to the guacamole. Serve traditionally with chips or, for a healthier option, slice up crunchy vegetables like jicama, carrots, and red pepper. Dig in!

CRAVING CHOCOLATE PROTEIN BARS

Craving the tastes of a decadent piece of gooey chocolate fudge? Satisfy your taste buds with all the flavors of a decadent dessert with this nutritious and delicious chocolate protein bar recipe. From a post-workout snack to an in-between-meals pick-me-up, you'll feel satisfied and energized with these tasty bars.

*Makes 12–16 bars

Ingredients

1 ½ cups fresh dates, packed & pitted

1 cup warm water (to soak dates)

1 cup cashews

1/3 cup old fashioned rolled oats (gluten-free if necessary)

¼ cup unsweetened shredded coconut

¼ cup all natural sweetened plant-based chocolate protein powder.

1/3 cup unsweetened cocoa powder or raw cacao powder

1 ½ tablespoons coconut oil, melted

1 teaspoon vanilla extract

¼–½ teaspoon sea salt

Method

Combine the dates and warm water in a small bowl. Let stand for about 5 minutes until dates are soft. Remove water and pat dry with paper towels. (If dates are already soft, skip this step.)

Place the cashew and oats in a food processor and process until finely chopped. Add the dates, protein powder, cocoa powder, melted coconut oil, coconut, vanilla, and salt. Process until the dates are finely chopped and blended and the mixture begins to stick together. Transfer the mixture to the lined loaf pan. It will be crumbly at first. Use parchment paper or wax paper on top of the bar mixture to pack and flatten the mixture evenly in the pan; leave the paper to cover. Refrigerate 1 hour or more until firm. Using the edges of the paper liner, lift the mixture from the pan and uncover. Cut into individual bars. Store in the refrigerator up to 5 days or freeze for longer-term storage.

Note: You can use any combo of nuts.

LEMON COCONUT ENERGY BITES

These tasty, sweet, and tangy energy balls are perfect just about any time you need a boost. With healthy fats from the coconut and cashews, plus a dose of plant-based protein, the delicious treats will help keep your blood sugar stable in between meals. Keep a stash in the freezer to have a satiated snack or dessert on hand always!

*Makes approximately 20 balls

Ingredients
1 cup cashews
1 packed cup Medjool dates, pitted
½ cup unsweetened shredded coconut, plus more to roll in
1 tablespoon maple syrup
2 tablespoons lemon juice
½ teaspoon vanilla
½ teaspoon sea salt
1 tablespoon lemon zest
Extra coconut for rolling

Method
Place the cashews in a food processor and pulse until crumbly, but not completely smooth. Next, add remaining ingredients except for the lemon zest. Process until the mixture is well-combined. Add in the zest and pulse for about 30 more seconds, until all the ingredients are incorporated. (It will be sticky.) If the mixture is too sticky to handle, place in freezer for about 15–20 minutes until firm enough to roll. Using a small spoon, scoop

out the mixture and roll into bite-sized morsels (about 1-inch), forming with your hands. Roll each ball in coconut. Place in the refrigerator on a baking tray for at least an hour before serving. Store any remaining energy balls in an airtight glass container up to 3 days in the refrigerator or freeze for one month. Enjoy!

MAMA ON THE GO TRAIL MIX

Trail mix is portable, customizable, and can be stored in the bottom of your diaper bag or handbag without any refrigeration necessary. Use this combination of nuts, seeds, and superfoods as inspiration, and then come up with your own variation.

*Makes 3 ½ cups

Ingredients
¾ cup almonds
½ cup walnuts
½ cup sunflower seeds
1 cup Goji berries
¼ cup raw cacao nibs
½ cup coconut flakes

Method
Mix all ingredients in a bowl and store in an airtight container.

VIBRANT VEGGIE SOUP

Filled with phytonutrients, this sumptuous soup is a great way to meet your vegetable requirement with just one bowl! Make a big batch on the weekend and then serve this soup alongside a meal, or enjoy it anytime as a snack to take the edge off in between lunch and dinner.

*Serves 8–10

Ingredients
1 yellow or sweet onion, diced
1 clove garlic, minced
4 carrots, chopped
3 celery stalks, chopped
2 tablespoons of high quality olive oil
4 cups vegetable broth
1-2 cups water, depending on desired thickness
1 28-ounce can diced tomatoes* (or if in season, equivalent of fresh tomatoes, chopped)
1 6-ounce container tomato paste*
1 ½ cups garbanzo beans, drained (if using canned, choose BPA-free)
6 cups vegetables, chopped (broccoli, red pepper, yellow squash, zucchini, green beans, cauliflower etc.)
2 tablespoons fresh herbs, chopped (parsley, oregano, and/or thyme)
1 teaspoon sea salt
3 cups fresh spinach leaves (reserve until the end)
Sea salt and pepper to taste
Red pepper flakes (optional for an additional kick)

*Due to the acid in the tomatoes and the possibility of BPA in cans, choose a carton or glass over canned when possible.

Method

Heat 2 tablespoons of olive oil in soup pot and add in onion, garlic, celery and carrots. Sauté until lightly browned then add in fresh herbs and sea salt to coat the vegetables. Next, add the vegetable broth, garbanzo beans, tomatoes, and tomato paste. Mix thoroughly and then place the chopped vegetables into the pot. Add enough water or additional broth to cover the vegetables. Bring the mixture to a boil, then reduce it to a simmer. Cover for about 35–40 minutes or until the vegetables are soft and can be pierced with a fork. Turn off the heat and add in 3 cups of fresh spinach leaves. Place the lid back on the pot for 5 minutes to allow the spinach to steam. Season with sea salt and fresh pepper to taste. Enjoy!

Works Cited

1   Deepak Chopra, David Simon, and Vicki Abrams, *Magical Beginnings, Enchanted Lives* (New York: Harmony, 2005), 7.

2   Eckhart Tolle, *The Power of Now: A Guide to Spiritual Enlightenment* (Vancouver: Namaste Publishing, 2004), 35.

3   David Ji, *The David Ji Blog*, accessed Month dd, yyyy, http://davidji.com/meeting-our-needs.

4   Chopra et al, *Magical Beginnings, Enchanted Lives*, 6.

5   Joshua Rosenthal, *Integrative Nutrition (Third Ed.): Feed Your Hunger for Health and Happiness* (Austin, TX: Greenleaf Book Group, LLC, 2007).

6   Mary M. Murphy, Nicolas Stettler, Kimberly M. Smith, and Richard Reiss, "Associations of consumption of fruits and vegetables during pregnancy with infant birth weight or small for gestational age births: a systematic review of the literature," *International Journal of Women's Health* 6, (2014): doi: 10.2147/IJWH.S67130

7   Michael Pollan, *Food Rules: An Eater's Manual* (New York: Penguin Books, 2009) 41.

8   "Executive Summary: EWG's 2016 Shopper's Guide to Pesticides in Produce," Environmental Working Group, 2016, May 14, 2016 https://www.ewg.org/foodnews/summary.php.

9   "Executive Summary: EWG's 2016 Shopper's Guide to Pesticides in Produce," Environmental Working Group, 2016, May 14, 2016 https://www.ewg.org/foodnews/summary.php.

10 Bill Sears, "Excitotoxins in Your Food," *Dr. Sears Wellness Institute* (blog), August 24 2015 https://www.drsearswellnessinstitute.org/blog/excitotoxins/.

11 Geneen Roth, *When You Eat at the Refrigerator, Pull Up a Chair: 50 Ways to Feel Thin, Gorgeous, and Happy (When You Feel Anything But)* (New York: Hachette Books, 1999)

12 Danny Penman, "The Chocolate Meditation," *Mindfulness in a Frantic World* (blog), September 12, 2011, https://www.psychologytoday.com/blog/mindfulness-in-frantic-world/201109/the-chocolate-meditation.

13 "Wheel of life," Act Now, accessed Month dd, yyyy, http://www.actnow.ie/resources/wheel-of-life.

14 "Why Gratitude Is Good." Robert Emmons, Greater Good. November 16, 2010, http://greatergood.berkeley.edu/article/item/why_gratitude_is_good

15 Louise Hay, *101 Power Thoughts (Abridged)* (Carlsbad: Hay House, 2004).

16 Mohandas K. Gandhi, *Gandhi: An Autobiography: The Story of My Experiments with Truth*, trans. Mahadev H Desai (Boston: Beacon Press, 1993).

17 "Prenatal Yoga: What You Need to Know," The Mayo Clinic, last modified December 15, 2015, http://www.mayoclinic.org/healthy-lifestyle/pregnancy-week-by-week/in-depth/prenatal-yoga/art-20047193.

18 Steven Campbell, *Making Your Mind Magnificent: Use the New Brain Science to Transform Your Life: End Negative Thinking, Improve Focus and Clarity, and Be Happier* (Rohnet Park: Intelligent Heart Press, 2014), 49.

19 "The Time that Matters Most," Marianne Williamson, Oprah.com, July 2008, http://www.oprah.com/spirit/Marianne-Williamson-The-Time-That-Matters-Most.

20 Gurmukh K. Khalsa, *Bountiful, Beautiful, Blissful: Experience the Natural Power of Pregnancy and Birth with Kundalini Yoga and Meditation* (NewYork: St. Martin's Griffin, 2004), 39.

21 Levine via Chopra

22 Khalsa, *Bountiful, Beautiful, Blissful*, 151.Gurmukh

23 Pam Grout, *E-Squared: Nine Do-It-Yourself Energy Experiments That Prove Your Thoughts Create Your Reality* (Carlsbad: Hay House Insights, 2012), 1-20.

24 Bruce Lipton, *The Biology of Belief,* (City: Publisher, Year).

25 "Six Basic Needs That Make Us Tick," Tony Robbins, *Entrepreneur.* December 4, 2014.

26 Khalsa, *Bountiful, Beautiful, Blissful,* 54.

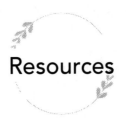

Resources

Self-Care Support Sheet

Use this sheet to write down your favorite go-to self-care tools. Hang or keep this sheet somewhere for easy access to help you in times when you need some guidance and support.

My favorite yoga postures: ex: <u>When my legs/ankles feel swollen, I do legs-up-the-wall pose.</u>

_____

_____

_____

Peace in the Present Moment: <u>Write down 3 things I'm grateful for in this moment.</u>

_____

_____

_____

My go to foods when I'm feeling nauseous:

_____

_____

_____

Affirmations to lift me up:

_____

_____

_____

When I'm feeling sad, lonely or down, I'll call or see this person/ these people:

_____

_____

_____

When my energy is low, I can:

_____

_____

_____

My favorite nutrient-dense snacks:

_____

_____

_____

If I've been neglecting my self-care, I can:

_____

_____

_____

My favorite ways to feel better and three lines

_____

_____

_____

Feel-Good Flicks

As Good as It Gets
Can't Buy Me Love
Chocolat
Clueless
Forrest Gump
Groundhog Day
Legally Blonde
Little Miss Sunshine
Midnight in Paris
Mr. Mom
Mrs. Doubtfire
My Best Friend's Wedding
My Fair Lady
Overboard
Pretty Woman
Shall We Dance
Something's Gotta Give
The Best Exotic Marigold Hotel
The Full Monty
The Holiday
The Hundred-Foot Journey
The Intern
The Princess Bride
Uncle Buck
Under the Tuscan Sun
When Harry Met Sally
You've Got Mail

Relaxing Music

This list offers a variety of relaxing music, including: Classical, Sitar, Instrumental, and Vocal. Listen to the songs to discover which leads to you a deeper sense of calm and relaxation. I've offered a favorite song or two from each album to help you get started.

Calm Baby by Phillip Kanakis
"Calm Baby" and "Untroubled"

Flying by Garth Stevenson
"Flying" and "Earth"

Grace by Snatam Kaur
"Long Time Sun"

Sanctuary of Rejuvenation by Aeoliah
"Angel Love"

Simply Baroque by Yo-Yo Ma
"Matthäus-Passion"

Sitar Secrets by Al Gromer Khan
"Caru Caru"

So Much Magnificence by Steve Gold
"There Is So Much Magnificence"

Unity by Sean Johnson & The Wild Lotus Band
"Nur Allah Nur"

Zen Master's Diary by Darshan Ambient
"A Day Within Days"

Mindfulness and Meditation Resources

Mindful Magazine
http://www.mindful.org/mindful-pregnancy/

Mindfulness for Pregnancy (App)
https://itunes.apple.com/us/app/mindfulness-for-pregnancy/

Headspace (Website and App)
"Health Pack" Pregnancy
www.headspace.com

Magical Beginnings, Enchanted Lives (Book)
By Deepak Chopra and David Simon

Meditations for Pregnancy (Book and CD/Audio)
By Michelle Leclaire O'Neill, Ph.D., R.N

Mindful Birthing (Technique)
www.mindfulbirthing.org

Hypnobirthing (Technique)
us.hypnobirthing.com

Prenatal Nutrition and Nutrient Dense Recipes

Beautiful Babies: Nutrition for Fertility, Pregnancy,
Breast-feeding, and Baby's First Foods
by Kristen Michaelis and Joel Salatin

Happy, Healthy Pregnancy Cookbook: Over 125
Delicious Recipes to Satisfy You, Nourish Baby, and
Combat Common Pregnancy Discomforts
by Stephanie Clarke and Willow Jarosh

Real Food for Mother and Baby: The
Fertility Diet, Eating for Two, and
Baby's First Foods
By Nina Planck

The Nourishing Traditions Book of Baby & Child Care
by Sally Fallon Morell and Thomas S. Cowan

The 100 Healthiest Foods to Eat During Pregnancy:
The Surprising Unbiased Truth about Foods You Should
be Eating During Pregnancy but Probably Aren't
by Jonny Bowden and Allison Tannis

Whole Food Energy: 200 All Natural Recipes to
Help You Prepare, Refuel, and Recover
by Elise Museles

Journal Page

Journal Page

Journal Page

Journal Page

Journal Page

Printed in the United States
By Bookmasters